OPERATION FIVE-STAR:

Service Excellence in the Medical Practice— Cultural Competency, Post-Adverse Events, and Patient Engagement

JAMES W. SAXTON, ESQ.

AND

MAGGIE M. FINKELSTEIN, ESQ.

CONTRIBUTING AUTHORS:
L. Greg Pawlson, MD, MPH, FACP and
Diane Pinakiewicz, MBA, CPPS

Foreword by Kevin Bingham, ACAS, MAAA

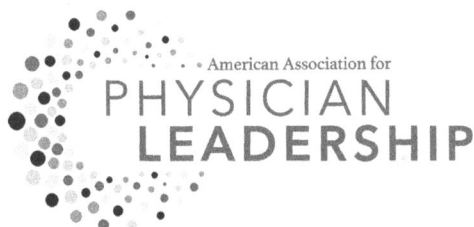

American Association for
PHYSICIAN
LEADERSHIP

AAPL books are available at special quantity discounts to use as premiums and sales promotions, or for use in corporate training programs. For more information, please write to Special Sales at journal@physicianleaders.org

This publication is designed to provide general information and is sold with the understanding that neither the author nor the publisher is engaged in rendering legal, accounting, ethical, or clinical advice. If legal or other expert advice is required, the services of a competent professional person should be sought.

13   8 7 6 5 4 3 2 1

Copyedited, typeset, indexed, and printed in the United States of America

PUBLISHER

Nancy Collins

EDITORIAL ASSISTANT

Jennifer Weiss

DESIGN & LAYOUT

Carter Publishing Studio

COPYEDITOR

Pat George

Table of Contents

Acknowledgments

First and foremost, we thank you, the reader, for your interest in this important topic and your commitment to five-star service excellence in healthcare. We hope that you find the content of this book helpful to your on-going pursuit of five-star service.

We also want to thank the many physician practices, physicians, practice managers, and staff members with whom we have worked over the years and who have let us into their practices to help them evaluate five-star service and to provide them with support to move up the five-star curve.

A special thank you to the various professionals who contributed to this text, including: Gary Kaplan, MD, FACP, FACMPE, FACPE; L. Gregory Pawlson, MD, MPH, FACP; Diane Pinakiewicz, MBA, CPPS; Steven Schwaitzberg, MD,; Richard Waldman, MD; Martha Dawson, RN, BSN; Mandy Foley, RN; Lois Summers; and Lisa Eng, DO.

We dedicate this book to our spouses—James' wonderful and talented wife, Sally, and Maggie's amazing husband, Andrew DiCostanzo—and to all the doctors that we are privileged to work with and represent every day.

We wholeheartedly thank Stevens & Lee and its leadership, who continue to support our Healthcare Litigation and Risk Management Group's vision, allowing us to innovate and help physicians, their practices, hospitals, and post-acute care facilities to not only defend professional liability claims, but also to help them mitigate professional liability risk in an ever-changing environment.

And of course, we extend very sincere thanks to Greenbranch Publishing and its team of talented professionals including Nancy Collins, Jennifer Weiss, Laura Carter and Patricia George.

JAMES SAXTON
MAGGIE FINKELSTEIN

About the Authors

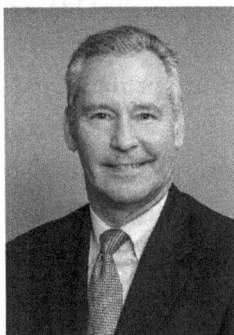

James W. Saxton has represented physicians and hospitals in state and federal courts for over 30 years. He is presently the chairman of Stevens & Lee's Health Care Litigation and Risk Management Group and co-chair of the firm's Health Care Department. His practice includes healthcare litigation and the representation of healthcare organizations and medical professional liability insurers. Mr. Saxton is a Fellow of the Litigation Counsel of America—a position reserved for less than one-half of 1% of the lawyers in the country.

Mr. Saxton uses his extensive expertise as a litigator to advise healthcare providers throughout the United States in connection with understanding and reducing their professional liability risk by promoting excellence in patient satisfaction and incorporating certain loss control and safety protocols. He develops risk-reduction strategies for medical professional liability insurers, hospitals, and health systems, as well as physician organizations, and has created tools and educational programs to support them.

Mr. Saxton is a prolific writer on the subject of reducing medical liability risks. He has published more than 200 articles, seven textbooks, and several handbooks. He also presents frequently to nationally prominent healthcare organizations on healthcare industry liability and risk issues. He has lectured at the American College of Surgeons, the American Society for Metabolic and Bariatric Surgery, the American Urology Association, the American Health Lawyers Association, the American Society for Healthcare Risk Management, and the Physician Insurers Association of America.

He is a Fellow of the College of Physicians of Philadelphia, past board member of the Surgical Review Corporation, and a board director of SE Healthcare Quality Consulting, LLC. He is a past chair of the American Health Lawyers Association's Healthcare Liability and Litigation Practice Group and was named to the American Health Lawyers Association's Accountable Care Organization Task Force. Contact James Saxton at jws@stevenslee.com.

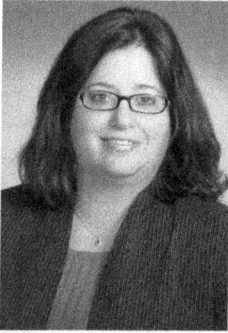

Maggie M. Finkelstein is a shareholder with Stevens & Lee's Health Care Litigation and Risk Management Group. She focuses her practice on helping physicians, hospitals, centers, clinics, and other healthcare providers reduce liability risk and enhance patient safety and quality of care.

Ms. Finkelstein has researched and developed risk mitigation opportunities for healthcare professionals nationwide in the areas of five-star service excellence, patient satisfaction, and post-adverse event communication. She has also evaluated specialty-specific liability risk in various medical specialties, including bariatric surgery, obstetrics, and gastroenterology. This research and evaluation led to the creation of medical professional liability insurance companies, which embed specialty-specific safety and risk management programs.

Most recently she has worked with leading clinical content experts to create new web-based quality dashboards for risk mitigation and to create specialty-specific patient experience of care survey content that are embedded into the insurance company. She also provides event management and risk mitigation advice, corporate guidance and support, oversight and implementation of the safety programs and education, and support in claims defense and management.

In addition, she works with a team of legal and clinical professionals to create safety companies that provide specialty-specific safety services, including SE Healthcare Quality Consulting and OB Consult. She serves as a project lead on significant quality and safety and peer review evaluations for academic medical centers, international medical centers, and community based hospitals.

Ms. Finkelstein regularly publishes articles, white papers, book chapters, and books on loss control, risk management, and related medical professional liability issues. She also presents online programming, including webcasts, and live, national programming on these same issues, for organizations such as the American College of Obstetricians & Gynecologists, Pennsylvania Health Care Association, and 2014 American Association of Gynecological Laparoscopists and for the Surgery Resident Program at the 2014 Clinical Congress of the American College of Surgeons.

She is a former law clerk for the Honorable William W. Caldwell, U.S. District Court for the Middle District of Pennsylvania, and is a registered patent attorney with the United States Patent and Trademark Office. Contact Maggie Finkelstein at mmf@stevenslee.com.

Contributors

L. Gregory Pawlson, MD, MPH, FACP, immediate past executive director for quality innovation for Blue Cross Blue Shield Association and past executive vice president of the National Committee for Quality Assurance, Washington, DC

Gary Kaplan, MD, FACP, FACMPE, FACPE, chairman and CEO, Virginia Mason Health System, Seattle, WA

Diane Pinakiewicz, MBA, CPPS, immediate past president of The National Patient Safety Foundation, Boston, MA

Lisa Eng, DO, member of the Medical Society of the State of New York's Committee to Eliminate Healthcare Disparities, Albany, NY

Steven Schwaitzberg, MD, chief of surgery, Cambridge Health Alliance, Cambridge, MA

Richard Waldman, MD, president of the medical staff, St. Joseph's Hospital Health Center, Syracuse, NY and past president of the American College of Obstetricians and Gynecologists, Washington, DC

Mandy Foley, RN, patient experience leader, Camden Clark Medical Center, Parkersburg, WV

Martha Dawson, RN, BSN, director of women's and children's services, Camden Clark Medical Center, Parkersburg, WV

Lois Summers, General Internal Medicine of Lancaster, Division of Physician's Alliance Limited, Lancaster, PA

Foreword

Chinese philosopher Lao Tzu once said, "A journey of a thousand miles begins with a single step." It's hard to believe that Jim and Maggie's focus on five-star customer service began over a decade ago. I can still remember reading their material and being inspired by the message they were sharing with others. To this day, I still cite their work when speaking at conferences and discussing the importance of communicating effectively and engaging patients.

Jim and Maggie's focus on bringing a five-star service culture from other industries sets the stage for healthcare professionals to improve their service excellence and event management skills. In 2007, Jim and I co-authored an article in *Physician Insurer Magazine* titled "Avoiding the Next Malpractice Crisis—Can We Shape Our Destiny?" We shared the following vision: "Perhaps, if physicians were able to deliver five-star customer service like Disney or The Ritz-Carlton, there would be fewer malpractice claims, and the outcome of successful claims would be less severe. Something like 'five-star customer service' would also foster an environment where physicians and hospitals learn from their mistakes, helping to prevent future errors. In other words, there would be a no-shame, no blame environment that encourages continuous quality improvement."

With the release of *Operation Five-Star: Service Excellence in the Medical Practice—Cultural Competency, Post-Adverse Events, and Patient Engagement,* I am proud to say that Jim and Maggie have taken further steps towards achieving this vision. In today's ever changing healthcare environment with the shift from volume to value, increased focus on patient experience and the power of social media, the number of stressors impacting physician practices and hospitals is on the rise. *Operation Five-Star* lays the foundation for reaching the elusive fifth star where customer excellence can truly set a physician practice apart from other practices. From the newest employee to the most tenured medical professional, Jim and Maggie discuss the interactions between doctors and staff (and the patients they serve) to drive five-star customer service into the DNA of the organization. Examples of such interactions include the patient's first contact with the practice (i.e., their "first impression"), answering calls, electronic medical records, communication between practitioners in front of patients, filling out forms, providing care, care plan adherence, addressing patient complaints, and post-adverse event communications.

At the end of the day, patients want to feel valued and cared about by their healthcare providers. Five-star organizations convey this feeling to patients through both the physician-patient relationship and the practice-patient relationship. When done right, patient engagement not only improves the practice and hospital environment, but favorably impacts performance-based payments tying reimbursements to quality outcomes and decreases the probability of a medical malpractice claim or state board complaint by reducing service lapses and miscommunications. In situations where an adverse event happens, a five-star culture allows physicians and patients to develop a trusting relationship that helps to transcend an adverse event. Most importantly, a trusting relationship improves the likelihood that patients and their families will return to the physician post-adverse event for answers instead of first reaching out to a plaintiff lawyer. Service lapses may not cause a medical malpractice claim, but it is important to recognize that plaintiff lawyers will happily leverage service lapses to inflame a jury and increase the value of a settlement or jury award.

I have had the pleasure of working with Jim and Maggie and have seen the impact their strategies have had on the healthcare clients we serve. Just as they inspired me over a decade ago, they continue to do so. Since first hearing their five-star customer service message, I have had Jim speak at my annual (Medical Professional Liability) MPL ExecuSummit Conference 8 times out of the past 10 years. The reason is simple . . . the passion Jim and Maggie have for this topic shines through in everything they do.

Henry Ford once said, "Quality means doing it right when no one is looking." I believe Jim and Maggie provide the insights in *Operation Five-Star* to help office practices and hospitals do it right whether patients are looking or not. From tips (e.g., 10 key communication tips, 58 five-star tips, etc.), preparation guidelines to powerful examples, their book sets the stage for healthcare organizations to achieve that elusive fifth star. Best of luck with your five-star journey and improving patient engagement in your healthcare practice!

KEVIN M. BINGHAM, ACAS, MAAA
Co-chair, Casualty Actuarial Society's Innovation Council
Advisory board member and Chairman of the annual MPL ExecuSummit

Past chairperson, Casualty Practice Council Medical Professional Liability
(MPL) Subcommittee

Official spokesperson for the American Academy of Actuaries in Washington

Regular contributor to *Physician Insurer Magazine, Claims Magazine,
Contingencies Magazine* and other publications on issues facing the
financial services and healthcare industries. To date, Mr. Bingham has
authored over 60 articles and spoken at over 100 conferences, seminars
and educational events

Glastonbury, Ct.

Introduction

In the past, five-star was perhaps one of the most underestimated concepts in the healthcare industry. Not anymore. Five-star customer service is something we all demand in our everyday lives—in our homes, businesses, and personal lives—and now it's becoming one of the cornerstones of healthcare delivery.

Its benefits are well-established, including:

- A better working environment;
- Increased staff retention;
- Higher patient satisfaction;
- Greater patient engagement leading to better outcomes;
- Reduced liability risk; and
- Positive economics.

The healthcare segment has made much progress, but there is still plenty of room for improvement. Five-star has taken on new importance, and medical practices throughout the country are refocusing and even doubling down on their efforts.

WHY A NEW BOOK ABOUT FIVE-STAR?

Plenty has been written about patient satisfaction. However, the new healthcare environment motivates us to re-energize this concept and brings us some new terms and a need to re-examine some age-old terms, like *patient centeredness*, *patient satisfaction*, *patient perception*, and *patient experience*. All of these concepts are driven by new aspects of five-star service excellence. Several of these new aspects deserve our attention:

- The patient experience;
- HCAHPS and CG-CAHPS surveying;
- The practice-patient relationship;
- Specialty-specific patient experience;
- True patient engagement;

- Post-adverse event communication as a part of the patient experience;
- Five-star service from the perspective of a practicing physician;
- Five-star service from the perspective of a health policy expert; and
- Cultural competency as part of patient experience.

Given the massive changes taking place for our doctors and patients, these five-star concepts are all the more important. Making sure we focus on how patients feel, understanding how their experience is affected by these changes, and getting behind their dis-satisfaction are all critical success factors. Attending to these areas not only can better prepare you and your practice for new reimbursement methodologies, but also reduce your medical professional liability exposure.

This book is based on research and data and discussions with national content experts as well as practitioners with front-line experience working at hospitals and in physician practices throughout the country. It includes a combination of clinical, health policy, legal, and patient perspectives of the patient experience. Most importantly, the information is meant to be practical and user-friendly—something you can use at your practice or hospital next week.

CHAPTER 1

What Is Five-Star Service, *Really?*

What is five-star? You know it when you experience it. We have all received five-star service and appreciate the difference.

Consider the restaurant industry or the lodging industry, where the five-star concept has its roots. You know what a five-star restaurant is when you dine there, and you know a five-star hotel when you stay there. Where it gets interesting is that many of you have received five-star service at a hotel that's been rated three-star and you've endured two-star service at a hotel that's touted as five-star. Why? It's because true "service" goes beyond a good meal or a well-appointed hotel room. It focuses on the entire experience: what is said, the body language, and even the service recovery when necessary.

Five-star service is a high level of service, but one that is thoughtful as well. Five-star focuses on quality and service at every phase of your patients' experiences and interactions with your practice—in person or by telephone. It is not just about how nice you are or how often you smile (although those are good starts). Simply put, five-star is a *pervasive* culture that is *consistently* applied internally to each other and externally to your colleagues and of course your patients and their families.

True five-star customer service in healthcare is rare, which creates a real opportunity for medical practices to move up the five-star continuum and differentiate themselves.

Five-star customer service may seem to be common sense to those first introduced to the concept; however, in reality, providing five-star customer service on a consistent basis can be extraordinarily difficult, particularly when the individual health professional or practice is under stress. Why? Because true five-star service addresses behaviors, actions, and reactions. Further, it is far easier to provide five-star service when the EMR is working, everyone shows up for work, it's sunny and 75°, and you don't have a medical malpractice lawsuit looming over your head! Unfortunately this rosy scenario is not always the case. How an organization operates under stress at the macro and micro levels is critical to the success of the organization; this is when the five-star "culture" kicks in.

Simply put, five-star is a *pervasive* culture that is *consistently* applied internally to each other and externally to your colleagues and of course your patients and their families.

So many times we hear comments like:

"Our scores are already in the top 20%; we are very good in the satisfaction area."

"The doctors in our practice have not been sued much ... clearly we are doing something right!"

"We just do not have the time to establish five-star service right now. We are going to focus on taking care of patients."

"Most everyone in the practice understands this ... well not Dr. Smith. That's just the way he is. But, he's a great doc."

There is a degree of reasonableness to each statement, but they all also miss the point to some degree. Do not be satisfied by being in the top 20%, particularly under the present scoring system. It is great that you have not been sued, but that is not the only goal. Focusing on taking care of patients is critical, and five-star service can be a component of providing high-quality care. Today's "great" doctor or today's "rock star" will excel at five-star service! This culture can really propel your practice to the top.

It would seem that this concept of high-quality customer service is yesterday's news, yet, five-star has not permeated most organizations. That's due in part to perceived barriers to attaining a five-star practice. So, one of your goals should be to identify the barriers and work to overcome them. In conducting hundreds of five-star practice evaluations over the years, we have identified some common barriers to success, including:

- Belief that being in the top 20% is good enough;
- Lack of true buy-in from leadership;
- Lack of an objective understanding of where a practice is on the five-star baseline;
- Belief but without a real plan for implementation;
- Providing a rallying "kick-off" but then neglecting to nurture the culture;
- Lack of consistent *training* on the basics;
- Failure to focus on what truly matters to patients;
- Practices keep the naysayers for too long;
- Lack of ongoing measurement;
- Lack of a true "service recovery" process;
- Champions become frustrated . . . and give up
- Disregard of stressors; and
- Failure to incorporate into employee interviews/evaluations/compensation metrics.

Let's review some of these in greater detail.

Contentment with Current Scores. We have heard from hospitals and practices that they rate in the top 20%, so their work is complete. This is a false sense of security. First, it is recognized that many present scoring systems are flawed. Many are not specialty-specific, are overly generic, or should be considered as just a baseline. Many practices, after specialty-specific testing, find there are significant opportunities for improvement. The point is that the fifth star is elusive. You have to keep chasing it.

The fifth star is elusive.
You have to keep chasing it.

Lack of Buy-In from Leadership. Physicians and non-physician leaders play a critical role in getting five-star service to be a *cultural phenomenon*. Five-star service is about what you do, not what you say you are going to do. Others will watch the leaders and learn from them. If you are a leader, this is your hill.

Lack of a True Objective Baseline. If you do not know where your practice is on the specialty-specific five-star baseline, you will not be able to deploy your resources effectively. Every practice should undergo an objective five-star evaluation and use the results to identify the areas of opportunity and formulate the practice's short-term and long-term goals. At the end of the day, most practices are not where they thought they were on the five-star scale. Gathering the data to find out where you are is a good and necessary first step.

No Real Plan for Implementation. If there is no plan, then there will be no real forward movement to affect the five-star culture. Everyone will just continue with the day-to-day routine they know. A plan should be created that includes immediate, short-term, and long-term goals, as well as timetables, responsibilities, and accountability. We recommend establishing a five-star committee that meets quarterly, with an agenda that assures the five-star concept is front and center. To get something done, someone must be responsible for the five-star committee being successful. More on this in Chapter 3.

Lack of a Cultural Infrastructure. We have seen many practices embark on a five-star initiative, only to fail because the critical cultural infrastructure necessary to nurture the five-star concept was not fully developed. The basic culture must be in place first, otherwise it is an uphill battle that will not take hold for the long-term. This infrastructure can be established by leadership buy-in; through educational programs such as "Developing Your Five-Star Service Culture" or "How to be Part of Your Practice's Five-Star Service Culture" or "Maintaining and Enhancing Your Five-Star Service Culture"; and by making it part of the operations of your practice. This could include describing the culture on your website, including training in your orientation programs, and making it part of your evaluations and your compensation system.

Lack of Training on the Basics. Staff cannot be simply told, "Next Monday we are starting a five-star program . . . get ready!" They need education on the basics of the five-star concept, including: what, why, and how. This basic information can evolve to more advanced education about topics such as defusing anger, dealing with the frustrated patient, improving body language, and showing empathy. These educational processes can take place with adult online learning, web-based programs, inservice programs, or a combination. Eventually, great educational topics will come out of your own patient experience data.

Failure to Focus on What Truly Matters to Patients. Most healthcare professionals do what they do because they want to provide quality care to others. Clearly, clinical care is paramount, but interpersonal relationships are a key as well. Research tells us what patients and families want most from their physicians: to provide confidence, empathy, humaneness, personalized care, respect, thoroughness, and directness.[1] Patients want their healthcare providers to make them feel valued and cared about. The five-star concept supports the conveyance of this feeling to patients throughout the practice.

The most powerful tool to better understand what your specific patients believe is important is to survey them. To really understand what they want, you need to know what they want from you as their physician, but also what they expect from your practice as a whole. The patient experience is more than the brief 10-minute examination by you; it includes the check-in procedure, the receptionist, the waiting room, the décor, the cleanliness of your facility, the nursing staff, and so on. Finding out how patients feel about these areas through scientifically crafted questions is a critical success factor today.

Keeping the Naysayers for Too Long. Even practices that take five-star service seriously put up with the naysayers for seemingly reasonable reasons; however, the naysayers can be like a virus that infiltrates your practice, infecting one person after another until the five-star service culture deteriorates and is no longer pervasive or habitual.

Naysayers come in more than one flavor. Some are complete eye rollers and that's an easy case. Others say the right things on occasion but neither buy-in nor contribute to your five-star culture. In fact, they almost look for opportunities to complain or point out why it's not working. These are more subtle but just as important to address.

When you put up with these people, you are sending a message that their behavior is acceptable. Of course, you should first try to help them, counsel them, and provide them with additional training. However, if their negativity persists, they need to move on. Be sure to follow your internal employment policies and procedures and relevant laws as you go down the path of potential discipline, and ultimately dismissal. Believe us, when one individual is let go for not participating in the practice culture, it is a message heard loud and clear throughout the entire practice!

Lack of a True Service Recovery Process or Lack of Use of an Existing Process. No five-star culture can exist without a true service recovery process. By "service recovery," we mean management of any service breakdown, such as late appointments, missed lab notifications, or missed orders. These may seem like little things to the practice, but they are big things to the patient!

Often practices do not incorporate a service recovery program, believing that it would be too time consuming; however, the opposite is true. When done right, a service recovery process can save time for the entire healthcare team. Service recovery has a huge delta. If you address it right, you can get right back in the game. If you ignore it, it can put a bull's-eye on your back. Have a service recovery policy and procedure in place that includes responsibilities for managing these matters. In the long-term this will create greater efficiencies.

Support your champions. Celebrate the change. It takes time and support.

Champions Get Frustrated . . . Give Up. Without the cultural infrastructure, investment in training, and ongoing support, and with the other barriers discussed, the true champions of the five-star movement can become frustrated and give up. If what they are doing is not appreciated by the practice, they decide it's no longer worth the effort. Support your champions. Celebrate the change It takes time and support.

Stressors Are Unrecognized or are not Addressed. Oftentimes, stressors go unnoticed, or worse yet, are noticed but not addressed. Stressors cannot always be eliminated, but they often can be acknowledged and tension reduced.

Change produces stress, and there are a number of significant changes occurring in the healthcare environment, beyond every day stressors, including:

- In many practices, volume of patients is growing, requiring more staffing
- Greater emphasis on physician collaboration across specialties, often without a platform;
- Introduction of the Accountable Care Organizations and unfamiliar changes in reimbursement methods;
- Broadened scope of practice for medical professionals;

- New mandated preventive care requirements along with the systems necessary to accomplish and track;
- New payment methodologies that change the focus of reimbursement from volume to value;
- Emphasis on electronic medical records and related communication strategies;
- Increased requirements for data collection and therefore resources to do so;
- The introduction of the patient portal and its implications;
- Changes in the work/life desires of physicians; and
- The continuation of a difficult litigation environment.

One or a few of these challenges may have been enough of a stressor, but several of these are occurring simultaneously! It just makes five-star service all the more important. Again, the key is to acknowledge them and manage them and concurrently build your culture.

CONCLUSION

So five-star is the pervasive (excellence even under pressure) and consistent (by every individual in the organization) effort to focus on what is important to the patient and the family. It can be exceedingly simple: Be empathetic, smile when appropriate. It can be challenging: same-day scheduling. Regardless, the payoff is immense.

Congratulations to those of you who have high scores in customer satisfaction. You clearly are champions and are well-poised to take your practice/your hospital to the next level. Do not slow down. Continue to ramp up and challenge yourself to truly find out, per specific specialty, what makes a difference to your patients and how they can be better engaged. This is an area in which we all have a lot of room to grow.

Reference

1. Bendapudi NM, Berry LL, Frey KA, Parish JT, Rayburn WL. "Patients' perspectives on ideal physician behaviors." *May Clin. Proc.* 2006 Mar; 81(3):338-44.

CHAPTER 2

Why the Five-Star Focus Post-2014?

Why focus on five-star service post-healthcare reform? The traditional citations and evidence still apply: Hickson and Levinson introduced pioneering research in late the 1990s/early 2000s that linked physicians' communication with patients to liability risk. Levinson showed that certain physician communication behavior is associated with fewer malpractice claims.[1] Hickson reported that poor communication is a primary factor leading patients to sue and has linked communication lapses and patient complaints to professional liability claims.[2]

More recent data confirmed that patients consider service and bedside manner to be important physician traits. In 2008, the *Annals of Family Medicine* published a study that revealed that after thoroughness, patients want to see a doctor who knows them well, to see a doctor with a warm and friendly manner, and to have a shorter waiting time for an appointment.[3] Further, in 2008, the American Board of Medical Specialties released results of a study in which patients ranked physician bedside manner and communication skills as primary factors in choosing a physician.[4]

In 2008, Saxton and Finkelstein, with others from Press Ganey, co-authored a research publication that further substantiated the liability connection and satisfaction connection to five-star service, confirming that severity lies in inadequate management of adverse events, service lapses, and communication failures among healthcare professionals, staff, and the patients they treat. They concluded as well that the "plus" factors are perhaps more of a driver of litigation than previously thought.[5] In other words, these issues (lack of adequate management of adverse events, service lapses, and miscommunication) directly influence whether patients or their families seek the services of a plaintiff's law-yer, whether a claim will be pursued, and, ultimately, what will happen in the courtroom. Accordingly, medical practices can reduce liability exposure through the use of certain patient satisfaction strategies that are genuinely incorporated into the culture of the practice in a pervasive manner.

This is a paradigm shift in patient care and reimbursement from volume to value provides healthcare professionals with a catalyst to implement the most effective processes and procedures possible into their practices and, relevant to this book, to enhance the patient experience in healthcare.

Prior to 2010 national healthcare reform, a number of private and public payors had already linked performance of patient satisfaction to pay-for-performance.[6] Then, the Affordable Care Act (ACA)[7] and related regulations encouraged Medi-care, Medicaid, and plans participating in exchanges to broaden implementation of performance-based payment by tying reimbursement to quality outcomes, including patient experience, using new approaches to payment, rewards, incentives, and penalties. This is a paradigm shift in patient care and reimbursement from volume to value provides healthcare professionals with a catalyst to imple-ment the most effective processes and procedures possible into their practices and, relevant to this book, to enhance the patient experience in healthcare.

The phrase *volume to value* is tossed around a great deal. What does that mean in practical terms? According to L. Gregory Pawlson, MD, MPH, FACP, whose experience includes director of the Institute for Health Policy, Outcomes and Human Values and senior associate vice president for health affairs at the George Washington University Medical Center; Executive Director, Quality Innovations, Blue Cross Blue Shield Association; and Executive Vice President of National Committee for Quality Assurance):

"In essence, it means moving from the assumption that 'more is better' to looking carefully at every service process and task and asking the question: 'Is this necessary and desirable for good patient care, and if so, what is the best AND most efficient way to do it?' It will also mean creating a strong focus on creating value for patients through, among other things, optimizing the patients' experience of care."

In addition to patient experience ratings as part of payment determination, it will also help drive the success of a practice because of greater transparency for purchasers and patient-consumers of care. This patient experience data is increasingly being used by the "consumer-patient" to help them select physicians and practices—in essence, to shop for their healthcare! Patient ratings of their experience of care with hospitals and physicians practices are becoming increasingly available to the public in various formats. For example, the Centers for Medicare and Medicaid (CMS) created a new physician comparison website in January 2011 where patient experience ratings are posted.[8] That website was enhanced in June 2013 with better search functions and other information to improve accuracy. In 2013, CMS posted Physician Quality Reporting System (PQRS) information from physician groups with 100 or more healthcare professionals (who also used the web-based interface reporting process in 2013); and, in 2014, CMS may post all physician quality reporting system measures submitted by practices through a web-based process.[9] Some physician practices are posting their own survey scores on their own websites.

Physicians have already been dealing with the impact of technology on their practice reputation, including rating websites and blogs. However, social media has taken this to an entirely new level. Patients are leaving feedback in all these areas, good or bad. For example, here is a post seen on the internet:

> I have been to see him on three occasions. All three times I waited well over 1 hour past my appointment time. On my last visit I waited almost 2 hours beyond the appointment time. The reason I was given for the delay ... so many people need to see a surgeon and he can't refuse them. Nice guys perhaps but my advise is show up at least an hour late and save yourself the wait!

It can be extremely difficult for physicians to get negative comments removed from these sites.

Therefore, while traditionally a good risk-management strategy, patient experience is taking on even greater importance to physician practices in marketing and reimbursement. This is true not only with regard to CMS, but also with employers and certainly health payors.

PATIENT EXPERIENCE SURVEYING SINCE NATIONAL HEALTHCARE REFORM

Hospitals are feeling the impact of this new reimbursement system through the Hospital Consumer Assessment of Healthcare Providers and Systems (HCAHPS)[10] process. The Patient Protection and Affordable Care Act (PPACA) includes HCAHPS among the measures to be used to calculate value-based incentive payments in the Hospital Value-Based Purchasing program. This began with discharges after October 1, 2012 (Fiscal Year 2013).[11] HCAHPS Patient Experience of Care scores account for 30% of a hospital's overall rating (the other 70% is based on 12 clinical measures). To fund the incentive payments, hospitals participating in the value-based purchasing program will see their base operating Diagnosis-Related Group (DRG) payments for each patient discharge reduced (1% FY 2013; 1.25% FY 2014; 1.5% FY 2015; 1.75% FY 2016; and 2% FY 2017 and thereafter). They will compete to "win" back any part of that reduction.

In December 2012, CMS disclosed the bonuses *and penalties* that hospitals incurred beginning in January 2013. About half of the hospitals (1,427) received a penalty. On August 2, 2013, CMS issued its final rule increasing the penalty up to 1.25% for Fiscal Year 2014.[12]

Why should a physician care what happens to hospitals? Two reasons:

1. Your hospital will require it.
2. The physician practice is next.

The penalty for hospitals is expected to increase over the next several years, reaching 2%. Because of the way the calculations are made, value and quality for hospitals are not stagnant initiatives. The thresholds will continue to rise, requiring hospitals to offer better value and quality in order to be among the leaders in this area. So not only will this topic be important to hospitals now, but on a consistent go-forward basis as well. Let's look at some reasons the hospital's focus in this area becomes important to physicians where hospital-based care is provided, whether or not the physician is employed by the hospital. First, a focus on the office-based physician.

Physicians and Patient Experience—Office-Based

There are many reasons for physicians to enhance their patients' experience at the office, but perhaps one of the more compelling reasons is that physician-office-based patient experience scores will be part of physician reimbursement. For the first time, patient satisfaction metrics were part of an annual compensation report by Medical Group Management Association,[13] revealing that 2% of primary care physician compensation is based on patient satisfaction metrics; 1% of specialists' compensation is based on patient satisfaction metrics. However, these numbers are growing. In today's healthcare environment, it is the edge that can help enhance market share; it also can lead to better outcomes, which is the focus of healthcare reimbursement now and in the future.

Office-based and physician-focused patient experience surveys are useful tools to help you understand *your* patients' perceptions. The most useful tools are those that go beyond the broad HCAHPS surveys so you can better understand the "why" and "why not" of your results, and also be able to react in response to those results, enhancing scores in a more real-time fashion.

One company, MedStatix,[14] has done just that: created evidence-based physician practice-focused patient experience surveys using mobile technology. One important aspect of their surveys that is unique in the marketplace is that they are specialty-specific patient experience surveys. For example, MedStatix provides surveys tailored specifically to obstetrics, as their patient experiences differ from those of an orthopedic patient. One study has already shown that patient satisfaction scores differ across specialties. Patel and colleagues studied patient satisfaction across specialties, concluding that Ob/Gyn patient satisfaction ratings were 55% higher than other specialties, all else being equal.[15] Further, the odds of patients being satisfied with their doctors' friendliness and caring was three times higher for Ob/Gyns.

Specialty-specific patient experience surveys provide practices with a much-needed, deeper understanding of their patients' experiences.

The key to affecting patient perceptions, however, is going beyond the survey. It is one thing to know what your patients' perceptions are; it is another to evaluate them and use that information to enhance your patients' experiences with you and your practice. Often it is the lack of attention in the latter process that prevents physician practices from truly benefiting from patient experience surveys and increasing patient satisfaction.

Hospital-Based Physicians and Patient Experience

The patient-experience concept is also relevant to physicians who are hospital-based, whether employed or part of a hospital medical group. Many hospitals are holding their staff and physicians accountable for service, communication, and behavior—all key elements of the patient experience. Below are some examples of how patient-centeredness is becoming part of the hospital–physician relationship:

Physician compacts

Hospitals are using physician compacts to re-engage medical staff in a collaboration of providing care to the community based on set values, which often include patient-centeredness concepts such as customer service, teamwork, communication, accountability, reliability, respect, and professionalism. Virginia Mason Health System in Washington state is the oft-cited example (https://www.virginiamason.org/workfiles/HR/PhysicianCompact.pdf, last accessed 9/11/14). Virginia Mason Health System created a physician compact and a leadership compact to address roles and responsibilities. These are reciprocal agreements between organizations and their physicians to ensure aligned expectations and mutual accountability.

In April 2014, we talked with Virginia Mason Health System Chairman and CEO Gary Kaplan, MD, FACP, FACMPE, FACPE. He has served in this capacity since 2000, serves on national patient safety and quality organizational boards, and has received numerous safety and quality awards, including being ranked #3 on Modern Healthcare's list of the 50 Most Influential Physician Executives in 2014. (This is the ninth time he's been included on this list.)

Dr. Kaplan embraced the idea of a physician compact for Virginia Mason Health System in 2001. As a new CEO, he knew that the conversation with the physicians needed to change in order to achieve the organization's strategic plan and vision. Before the safety and quality movement and before consolidation, he wanted to substantively change the organization, anticipating coming change. He needed a way to bring the physicians on-board with the concepts in order to succeed—for the health system to survive into the future. So he wanted to re-establish a new deal and rules of engagement between the organization and its physicians.

His first step was to facilitate a physician retreat. He invited Jack Silverson, a pioneer in applying the social compact literature in healthcare, which led to the desire to create this new physician compact.

Dr. Kaplan explained: "The compact is a *reciprocal* agreement. It is not a job description for doctors. It sets forth what the physicians have the right to expect from the organization, and vice versa."

Dr. Kaplan explained: "The compact is a *reciprocal* agreement. It is not a job description for doctors. It sets forth what the physicians have the right to expect from the organization, and vice versa." He wanted to move his organization from the old model of physicians working in silos with autonomy to one focused on team-based care, which would enhance patient care, enhance efficiencies, and remove waste from care.

He formed a group of front-line physicians to serve as the "compact committee." That committee worked diligently for more than a year to get to an agreement that they all agreed with—every doctor in the system reviewed the compact. That same compact exists today.

The compact is used:

- In the hiring process. Dr. Kaplan provides the compact to every physician candidate who expresses interest in joining its medical group. His experience has been that about 95% of those like it; while about 5% say that they are not sure they want to be part of a culture that clear.
- In job descriptions.
- In performance management.
- For performance evaluation. The doctors and organization are held accountable. For example, if a physician strays from the compact, with repeated disruptive behavior, progressive discipline could be initiated to bring the provider closer to compact behavior.

Dr. Kaplan believes that the organization would not be where it is today without the compact. It is very, very well-received internally and is an important part of everyday at Virginia Mason Health System.

He noted that Virginia Mason Health System has compact**s**. While their physician compact gets the most recognition and notoriety, their process included creating a leadership compact. He recommends that facilities consider creating both.

While Dr. Kaplan is aware of some other health systems that created a physician compact, as he is often consulted, few hospitals have done so. Cedars-Sinai successfully incorporated a physician compact, impacting CMS core measures favorably and successfully installing health records into the system (after a previous fail prior to the physician compact process).

Dr. Kaplan noted that the content of the compact itself is important, but the *process* of creating that content is the most significant because it is the deep conversations that occur during the process that really make a huge difference, providing more transparency upfront about what the expectations.

When it comes to five-star service, patient experience is one of his health system's key pillars. They have a five-year patient experience plan that includes mandatory patient experience training for all staff, including physicians, and mandatory respect for people training. They regularly review and evaluate their HCAHPS scores as they are distributed, and have succeeded in having 50% of all their providers within the 90th percentile or above for patient satisfaction.

Remember, Virginia Mason Health System accomplished this *change* before the impetus that exists now. It is a proven strategy that can enhance the safety culture and the teamwork, and five-star service can be a component. The concept will continue to gain recognition in today's post-ACA environment, where reimbursement is increasingly tied to value and not volume, requiring hospitals to integrate physicians in a collaborative care delivery model focused on patient safety and quality of care, while also enhancing the patient experience of care. See Figure 2-1 for a sample physician compact.

Interviewing

The University of Washington Medical Center pairs patients with a clinical nurse specialist while interviewing prospective Ob/Gyn residents. The patients are provided with an evaluation tool that includes patient-centered interview questions.[16] While this example deals with residents, it is a trend that can be

PHYSICIAN COMPACT

Shared vision: It is our vision that physicians, staff, and leadership will be transparent in communication and planning, resulting in mutual respect, optimism, and cooperation within the entire organization. This Compact presents a framework of expectations regarding daily interactions and the creation of future policies and procedure. It is also our vision that through this process, our organization will create a "patient first" culture.

Physicians and Organization Leadership Commit to Each Other:
- Put aside all past conflicts and seek to understand all points of view in order to pursue progress
- Participate in the design and implementation of best clinical practices
- Communicate and participate in improving patient centered care
- Commit the resources to a sustainable culture of safety
- Support the shared vision

Organization's Commitment to Physicians:
- Be responsive in management decisions
- Commit to supporting an infrastructure for outcome measurement, patient experience measurement, and best practices in clinical and risk management
- Listen and communicate:
- Provide an infrastructure to support clinical integrity and global accountability
- Foster a team environment
- Embrace innovation

Physician's Commitment to Organization:
- Focus on patients first
- Enhance physician-patient relationship
- Acceptance of best clinical practices
- Commitment to a culture of team work
- Provide measurable quality care
- Participate in peer review
- Listen and communicate
- Be respectful of colleagues, staff, and patients and their families
- Participate in and use electronic medical record system and other technological advances

Signature of Physician: _____

Signature of Organization: _____

Figure 2-1. Physician Compact

expected to continue and to transcend into other evaluation and hiring settings in the hospital.

Education

Hospitals are educating their physicians on HCAHPS, including providing background information on HCAHPS, reviewing the questions pertinent to physicians, and training in those specific HCAHPS areas that reflect patient perceptions of physicians.[17] Other hospitals are concentrating on physician leadership training.[18] And the more progressive hospitals and health systems are focusing on the patient experience beyond HCAHPS requirements.

Peer review

Hospitals such as Methodist Health System[19] are tying back the education and patient satisfaction to the peer review process.

According to L. Greg Pawlson, MD, HCAHPS should be important to physicians for the following reasons[20]:

1. First and foremost, the issues reported in HCAHPS are important, according to patients. HCAHPS gauges how patients felt about their hospital stay in terms of areas that have been shown in research to be important to them, including whether they were treated with respect and compassion during their stay; if they felt they were listened to by all staff, including physicians; and if they received the information they needed at discharge. Some of these parameters also have been shown to have an impact on patient outcomes, including readmissions.

2. Several questions on HCAHPS directly reflect on medical staff conduct, including questions about how well staff members explained things and how well patients felt staff members listened.

3. Physicians' reputations can be enhanced or diminished by how well the hospital they use is viewed by the public; not only in terms of its technical performance, but also in how well it is able to meet patient expectations.

4. Finally, there is an increasing use of information by employers, payors, and patients related to performance, with HCAHPS being an important element for hospitals. Moreover, many pay-for-performance programs, which can affect hospital income and incomes of physicians employed by the hospital, are being linked to high performance on CAHPS surveys.

	HOSPITAL	NEW YORK AVERAGE	NATIONAL AVERAGE
Patients who reported that their nurses "Always" communicated well	70%	75%	79%
Patients who reported that their doctors "Always" communicated well	76%	77%	82%
Patients who reported that they "Always" received help as soon as they wanted	52%	61%	68%
Patients who reported that their pain was "Always" well controlled	61%	67%	71%
Patients who reported that staff "Always" explained about medicines before giving it to them	58%	59%	64%
Patients who reported that their room and bathroom were "Always" clean	67%	69%	73%
Patients who reported that the area around their room was "Always" quiet at night	55%	51%	61%
Patients who reported that YES, they were given information about what to do during their recovery at home	75%	83%	85%
Patients who gave their hospital a rating of 9 or 10 on a scale from 0 (lowest) to 10 (highest)	56%	63%	71%
Patients who reported YES, they would definitely recommend the hospital	57%	65%	71%

Figure 2-2. Sample Hospital Compare Chart

The focus on hospital-based patient experience should be important to physicians also, because it affects physician success. Interests of the hospital and physician are truly aligned in this area. For example:

1. Professional liability risk. Patient satisfaction is tied to liability risk[21], and experience shows that when a physician is named in a suit, the hospital is also often named as a defendant, and vice-versa. So, enhancing the patient satisfaction and experience in the hospital also reduces the frequency and

severity of lawsuits for hospitals and doctors. HCAHPS queries of patient perception include some areas of known liability risk such as:

- Patient understanding of discharge instructions and post-hospital-stay care; and
- Patient understanding of medication.

Both of these areas can involve patient non-compliance, which ties back to the very question queried by HCAHPS: Do patients understand the discharge instructions, post-discharge care needed, and medication? When they do not, it affects patient outcomes, which affects liability risk. Coordination and collaboration by hospitals and physicians in these areas can have a positive effect on liability risk.

2. Hospital competition. Armed with the publicly available information from HCAHPS, patients or consumers will have more information on which to base their decisions about where to receive hospital care when a choice is available. It stands to reason that all else being equal, patients will choose the hospitals with the higher patient satisfaction scores. When patients are attracted to a hospital, the physicians practicing at that hospital benefit as well. The nursing home industry especially has seen this trend of the impact of resident satisfaction scores, publicly available, on patient perceptions and choice of provider.[22] (See Figure 2-2.)

3. "Attractiveness" of physicians. This is an important new concept. You, as a physician, want to be attractive not just to patients (although that is important), but to hospitals, ACOs, and payors as well. Patients' perceptions of their experiences with the physicians at hospitals are evaluated by HCAHPS, and it is in the hospital's best interest to assure it credentials and/or hires physicians who exhibit the behaviors best-suited to enhance patient experience scores. As noted above, hospitals are beginning to use patients in the interviewing processes, evaluating patient-centeredness behaviors. The more patient-centered a physician is, the more attractive he or she will be to a hospital.

Physician "attractiveness" is becoming more important in today's environment where ACOs or ACO-like organizations are being created, as well as the Patient-Centered Medical Home and related neighborhood. The concept of collaboration among and within specialties and across settings is part of the embedded neighborhood concept, and this concept fosters shared accountability[23]

CONCLUSION

In healthcare, the five-star service excellence concept has traditionally been touted as a method of reducing professional liability risk for physicians and hospitals. That impact remains important; however, due to changes in the way healthcare is being delivered and reimbursed, the five-star service excellence concept has become a true critical success factor.

Realistically, this concept can concurrently reduce your medical professional liability exposure in a significant way and better one's economic performance. This is on top of creating a better environment in which to work. The time has never been better to, in a serious way, reintroduce this concept into your practice. The setting does not matter; it is critically important to all. Let's get started.

References

1. Levinson W, Roter DL, Mullooly JP, Dull VT, Frankel RM. "Physician-patient Communication: The Relationship with Malpractice Claims Among Primary Care Physicians and Surgeons." *JAMA.* 1997; 277: 553–559.

2. Hickson G, et al. "Patient Complaints and Malpractice Risk." *JAMA.* 2002; 287(22): 2951–2957; Hickson GB, Clayton EC, Githens PB, Sloan FA. " Factors that Prompted Families to File Malpractice Claims Following Perinatal Injury." *JAMA.* 1992; 287:1359–1363.

3. Sudeh Cheraghi-Sohi et al., *"What Patients Want From Primary Care Consultations: A Discrete Choice Experiment To Identify Patients' Priorities", 6 Ann Fam Med 107 (2008).*

4. *Bedside Manner, Board Certification Matter: Survey Reveals Top Qualities for Consumers Choosing a Doctor,* American Board of Medical Specialties, Aug. 4, 2008. (See http://www.abms.org/News_and_Events/news_archive/release_ABMS_Consumer_Survey.aspx.)

5. Saxton JW, Finkelstein MM, Bavin SA, Stawiski S. Reduce Liability Risk by Improving Your Patient Satisfaction. White Paper, South Bend, IN: Press Ganey; 2010.

6. Stawiski S, Bravin S, Fulton B. "The Impact of Patient Satisfaction on Pay-For-Performance in Medical Practices." (2008) (accessible at http://www.pressganey.com/Documents_secure/Medical%20Practices/White%20Papers/Med_Practice_P4P_6-08.pdf)

7. Patient Protection and Affordable Care Act (PPACA), Pub.L. No. 111-148, 124 Stat. 119 (2010).

8. www.medicare.gov/find-a-doctor/provider-profile.aspx . HCAHPS patient perception survey comprises 27 questions for discharged patients, about a recent hospital stay. Within those 27 questions are 18 core questions in the following areas of: 1) Communication—with nurses and doctors; 2) Responsiveness—of hospital staff; 3) Environment—cleanliness and quietness of hospital; 4) Pain management; 5) Communication—about medications and discharge information

9. *See* Fiegl C. "AMA pushes for more accurate Medicare Physician Compare." *AMEDNEWS.* (8/5/13) (last accessed 9/27/13) and accessible at http://www.amednews.com/article/20130805/government/130809985/6/?utm_source=nwltr&utm_medium=heds-htm&utm_campaign=20130805.

10. HCAHPS: Patients' Perspectives of Care Survey. Centers for Medicare and Medicaid Services, Baltimore, MD. 2012. Available from: https://www.cms.gov/HospitalQualityInits/30_HospitalHCAHPS.asp (last accessed March 15, 2012).

11. Patient Protection and Affordable Care Act (PPACA), Pub.L. No. 111–148, § 3024, 124 Stat. 119 (2010).

12. See CMS final rule to improve quality of care during hospital inpatient stays: Fact Sheet (8/2/13) (accessible at http://www.cms.gov/Newsroom/MediaReleaseDatabase/Fact-Sheets/2013-Fact-Sheets-Items/2013-08-02-3.html) (last accessed 9/12/14).

13. See Press Release: MGMA Survey: Physician compensation includes quality and patient satisfaction components (6/12/13) (accessible at http://www.mgma.com/about/mgma-press-room/press-releases/physician-compensation-includes-quality-and-patient-satisfaction-component) (last accessed 9/12/14).

14. *ROI HealthPartners* principals created a web-based patient experience survey platform. Its principals have a history of patient and customer satisfaction research surveying for Pharma and other industry (Fortune 100 companies). Their website is www.ROIHealthPartners.com.

15. Patel I, Chang J, Srivastava J, et al. "Patient satisfaction with obstetricians and gynecologists compared with other specialties: analysis of US self-reported survey data." *Patient Relat. Outcome Meas.* 2011 July; 2:21-26.

16. Profiles of Change: University of Washington Medical Center. Institute for Patient- and Family-Centered Care. Available from: http://www.ipfcc.org/profiles/prof-uwmc.html (last accessed September 27, 2013).

17. *See e.g.* Summa Health System (www.summahealth.org).

18. *Id.*

19. HCAHPS Background and Key Messages for Managers. Methodist Health System. Available from: http://www.methodisthealthsystem.org/documents/Medical%20Staff/HCAHPS%20Key%20Messages.pdf (last accessed January 10, 2014).

20. Commentary from L. Greg Pawlson, received by the authors on Nov. 22, 2013.

21. Saxton JW, Finkelstein MM, Bavin SA, Stawiski S. "Reduce Liability Risk by Improving Your Patient Satisfaction", Press Ganey, (2010): 1-11; Stelfox HT, Gandhi TK, Orav EJ, Gustafson ML. "The Relation of Patient Satisfaction with Complaints Against Physicians and Malpractice Lawsuits." *Am. J. Med.* 2005 Oct; 118(10):1126-33; Hickson GB, Federspiel CF, Pichert JW, Miller CS, Gauld-Jaeger J, Bo P. "Patient Complaints and Malpractice Risk." JAMA. 2002; 287:2951-57; Hickson GB, Clayton EC, Githens PB, Sloan FA. "Factors that Prompted Families to File Malpractice Clams Following Perinatal Injury." JAMA. 1992; 287:1359-1363; Levinson W, Roter DL, Mullooly JP, Dull VT, Frankel RM. 1997. Physician-patient Communication: The Relationship with Malpractice Claims Among Primary Care Physicians and Surgeons. *JAMA.* 277: 553-559; Beckman HB, Markakis KM, Suchman AL, Frankel RM. 1994. The doctor-patient relationship and malpractice: lessons from plaintiff depositions. *Arch Int Med.* 154(12): 1365-70.

22. *See e.g.,* Nursing Home Compare. Centers for Medicare and Medicaid Services, Baltimore, MD. (http://www.medicare.gov/NHCompare/Include/DataSection/Questions/SearchCriteriaNEW. asp?version=default&browser=IE%7C8%7CWindows+7&language=English&defaultstatus=0&pa gelist=Home&CookiesEnabledStatus=True (last accessed March 16, 2012)).

23. A Position Paper of the American College of Physicians. "The Patient-Centered Medical Home Neighbor: The Interface of the Patient-Centered Medical Home with Specialty/Subspecialty Practices." (2010). (Available from American College of Physicians, 190 N. Independence Mall West, Philadelphia, PA 19106) .

CHAPTER 3

You Must Have a Plan

Many practices, particularly in today's environment, understand the need to push their practice up the five-star customer service continuum, but ask the question, "How do we do it?" A roadmap for implementation of *five-star* customer service is essential for success in creating a sustainable *five-star* culture. The following provides the basics, and gives you a place to start, or in many cases, a plan to re-energize.

STEP 1: OBTAIN LEADERSHIP BUY-IN

A five-star program will not be sustainable without a commitment from the top of an organization. Perhaps you're the leader of the practice, or the non-physician CEO. Begin your efforts at the next administration/management meeting and present your pitch, including the empirical support for such an incentive. Be prepared to hear that the group is already providing five-star service! Challenge the conclusions. Ask for the specialty-specific surveys and the benchmarking data—the data may tell a different story. Leadership buy-in and leading by example will set a solid foundation for forward movement in understanding the concept and how important it is to the practice. This should not be hard, as the present business case for pursuing five-star service is powerful.

Once initial support is in place, the stage is set to begin building an infrastructure.

STEP 2: ESTABLISH A FIVE-STAR COMMITTEE

Changing a culture often begins with assembling champions. Create a five-star committee that includes some of these champions—people who understand and support the concept and exemplify it every day. Committee members should also include representatives from the entire spectrum: physicians, management, and staff. The committee's work need not be overly labor-intensive. The committee could meet four times a year, reviewing survey results and initiatives and suggesting the inservice programs. This keeps the topic of five-star service in front of the practice and helps prevent it from becoming just another agenda item. The committee owns it and becomes its champion.

The job of the committee is to execute the five-star plan, provide accountability, gather and evaluate data, guide improvement opportunities and "fixes," keep the focus, and make sure that internal and external issues are being addressed.

> **You do not have to call it the Five-Star Committee; it can be a Service Excellence Committee, Performance Improvement Committee, Patient Experience Committee. The name doesn't matter; what does matter is that it becomes one of your most important committees.**

Plan for your first five-star committee meeting, as an organizational meeting, bringing the entire committee together to pursue one vision. You do not have to call it the Five-Star Committee; it can be a Service Excellence Committee, Performance Improvement Committee, Patient Experience Committee. The name doesn't matter; what does matter is that it becomes one of your most important committees. The committee should set goals and prepare the basics: mission statement, value statement, employee promise, and three steps of service. The first meeting may be simply a resurrection of an existing committee, bringing new energy to an already-existing initiative.

Mission Statement. A mission statement can range from a simple one-sentence statement to a paragraph, with or without bullet points. Its purpose is to convey (without flowery speech or jargon) the reason(s) the organization or individual exists—its purpose for being, who it serves, how it will go about doing so (what the business is), and sometimes, what values guide/will guide the organization or individual in accomplishing the first two items.

Here's an example of a mission statement:

"It is the mission of All About You Medical Practice to provide our community with high-quality medical care, customized to the needs and values of our patients, and to create a relationship with our patients, enabling them to be a partner with us in their healthcare."

It is important to get the mission statement in front of your patients, employees, vendors, and management so all stakeholders understand that service excellence is part of the mission of the practice.

Values Statement. Values statements describe how the practice views key factors of service, including quality, service excellence, respect, trust, communication, and teamwork. The statements describe what practice members are striving for and how they view the importance of these aspects of service. For a medical practice, consider the values statement illustrated in Figure 3-1 (next page).

Employee Promise. The first committee meeting is also the time to set an employee promise so that they understand the corporate commitment to employee satisfaction. Many great service organizations have one, including Ritz Carlton. An example in healthcare could look like this:

"At (practice name) our employees are the most important resource in our service to patients. We promise to invest resources to support employee satisfaction, including:
- Being open to new and better ideas;
- Recognizing and rewarding contributions;
- Anticipating and responding to change;
- Providing needed technology and information; and
- Providing career growth opportunities.

We also promise to treat every employee as an equal and with respect."

Three Steps of Service. In addition, your five-star committee should identify "three steps of service" that define the core critical aspects of service for your practice. Example:
- A warm smile with every patient encounter.
- Active listening to foster understanding and cooperation, and reduce conflicts.

Our Values at _____
(Insert Name of Practice)

Quality & Safety: We strive to exceed standards for quality and safety as established in the healthcare industry. We are constantly evaluating and benchmarking for improvement in what we do.

Service Excellence: We strive to exceed the expectations of those we serve, including our patients, their families, and our colleagues in this and other practices and organizations with whom we work.

Respect: We recognize the uniqueness of all individuals and strive to be respectful and considerate of ethical, cultural, psychological and social preferences.

Trust: From the first moment our patients contact us, our patients know that they are a focal point of our attention. With every interaction, we try to demonstrate our care and concern for each one as an individual.

Communication: We strive for open and honest communication with our patients and among our peers. We want to create an environment that encourages an open dialogue and questions.

Teamwork: We genuinely care for and support those with whom we work. We know that we are more successful when we work together to achieve a common goal. We take pride in our workplace and take responsibility for making it a place we enjoy.

© 2014 Stevens & Lee

Figure 3-1. Sample Values Statement

- Effective communication skills and strategies.

On an on-going basis, the five-star committee should be tasked with:
- Re-evaluating the initial plan;
- Overseeing the execution of the five-star plan;
- Establishing timelines and content for educational programs and surveys;
- Gathering and evaluating five-star data (claims, surveys); and
- Incorporating and publishing the five-star "fixes."

With the plan in place, it is time to let your staff know all about it! This is a crucial aspect of this process. Your staff is a big part of making your five-star initiative successful.

STEP 3: KICK-OFF YOUR FIVE-STAR CULTURE PROGRAM TO STAFF

With the leadership on-board, the five-star committee working, and the basics in place, it is time to kick off the organizational commitment to five-star to the staff. Here are some examples:

1. Give the staff a written announcement from the organization's leader that explains what five-star service is and why your practice/group/department is implementing it. Make it sound as important and positive as it actually is. Make sure the announcement is signed by the leader.
2. Have a kick-off event. Have a dinner meeting, have a breakfast meeting, have a speaker, use a web-based educational program—it all works as long as your leaders are educated and engaged.
3. Share your vision with the staff and discuss their involvement.
4. Get your staff's five-star commitment to providing five-star service.

Make five-star service an operational part of your practice. Include it in your recruiting, interviewing for physicians and staff, part of evaluations and compensation. Figure 3-2 shows a sample Five-Star Service Excellence Attestation Document that you can use in this process.

A helpful hint: Make sure the physicians set the stage by demonstrating their own commitment to five-star service.

A helpful hint: Make sure the physicians set the stage by demonstrating their own commitment to five-star service. In one practice, one of the physicians who often started his hours later than the rest, told the staff that he would be starting on time and then changed his personal schedule so he arrived and started on time, consistently. Another physician went out of her way to say good morning to staff and complimented employees for the good job they were doing. Another doctor, who had relationship issues that overflowed into the office, mended fences. These simple acts created a buzz in the office. What a great lead off for their five-star introduction!

Five-Star Service Excellence

_____ is a practice committed to Five-Star Service Excellence. We want to create the best possible environment for our patient care, our physician(s) to practice, and our employees to work.

Our Five-star service is guided by the following principles:

- **First Impressions**—Know that with each encounter you create a first impression. Greet people with kindness and respect; have a professional appearance; and use proper telephone etiquette.
- **Professional & Effective Communication**—Communicate with a positive attitude to project confidence, elicit trust, and inspire excellence. Be aware of how you project verbally and non-verbally.
- **Ownership**—Take pride in what you do and be responsible for the outcomes of your efforts. Recognize that your work is a reflection of you and of _____.
- **Care & Respect**—Create pride and joy in the work place and a five-star environment for our patients, their families, employees and physicians. Respect the individuality of those you encounter.
- **Teamwork**—Act with integrity and be a positive ambassador for _____. Offer assistance and anticipate the needs of patients, their families, and co-workers.

To partner with _____ a personal commitment to our values and principles of Five-Star Service Excellence is required. As a member of this organization, my signature below attests to my beliefs in those values and principles.

_____   _____

Signature   Date

© 2014 Stevens & Lee

Figure 3-2. Five-Star Service Excellence Attestation Statement

Step 4: Set a one-year, three-year, five-year plan.

After the kick-off and implementation of the strategies described in the previous chapter, you should prepare a plan that allows for incremental implementation of specific five-star service strategies. Some areas may require a short-term to impact, while others may take longer. Your five-star committee should identify the short- and long-term goals, and evaluate them, and readjust them yearly. Here, we focus on the first year . . . assuring that the foundation is in place for maximum success in five-star service culture integration. Physicians and staff will need tools and strategies to succeed. The tools and strategies are based on the areas of need identified in the survey process.

We conducted a five-star service survey of over 500 physician practices, evaluating five-star service in physical design, examination/office visit, check out, human resources, telephone etiquette, and general service excellence. The following are examples of areas that needed improvement:

Telephone Etiquette. The telephone raises many customer service issues. Five-star service demands courteous discussions, prompt responses, and easy-to-understand telephone prompts. Practices can provide a telephone etiquette and scripting tool (Figure 3-3, below). Make sure team members smile into the phone.

Service Excellence: Telephone Etiquette Tips

First Impressions is the first component of Five-Star Service Excellence. A patient's first encounter with your practice will likely be by telephone. The patient's experience with your telephone system or your receptionist may very well establish the patient's perception of your practice.

The following recommendations are made to assist you in capturing a positive "First Impression:"
- Keep automated voice systems to less than 6 prompts;
- Early in an automated message, incorporate instructions to call 911 if the caller is experiencing a medical emergency;
- Provide patients with an information sheet about your telephone system;
- Provide background music or other recorded information while on hold;
- Provide training and education to employees addressing use of the telephone system and leadership expectations regarding telephone etiquette;
- Periodically evaluate your system using patient and employee feedback, and make changes accordingly;
- Make sure your recorded information is up-to-date;
- Periodically audit employees' telephone skills.

Telephone Etiquette Training Tips:
- Calls must be answered within 3 rings.
- Greet caller, identify your department and yourself.
- Say "May I help you" or "How may I help you."

(Continued next page)

- Do not eat, drink, or chew gum when on the phone.
- Speak slowly and clearly. Exude confidence, competence and care.
- Ask for permission of callers before putting a caller on hold.
- Explain delays to the caller on hold by getting back on the line every 30-40 seconds. Continue to check if the person would like to continue to hold or leave a message.
- When taking a message, repeat the call back number and the message.
- Return calls and answer messages within one business day.
- Make a good "last" impression. Ask if there is anything else that you can do for the caller and thank them.

Sample Script/Behavior Points:

"Good morning/afternoon, Dr._____ office. My name is_____. How may I help you today?"

"I'm sorry, _____ is unavailable right now. May I leave him/her a message that you called?"

"I'm sorry, _____ is on another call right now, would you like to hold for a few moments?"

"Thank you for holding Mr./Mrs./Ms./.Miss_____. I can put you right through to _____now."

Figure 3-3. Telephone Etiquette and Sample Script

Office Visit. A majority of practices were sensitive to how they greet patients and how they keep their healthcare information confidential. However, practice recommendations included reviewing patient wait times annually with an audit tool (Figure 3-4, below), setting patient expectations on the wait time, and ensuring all staff wear nametags (some states require it).

Wait Time Audit Tool

This tool can be used when auditing patient waiting times. It is divided into cycles to better identify where delays may be occurring. This will facilitate driving focused improvement efforts.

This tool can be placed on top of the patient's chart or on a clipboard and completed by staff during the various stages of the patient visit.

Cycle 1* can be initiated by the front desk staff, with the individual escorting the patient to the examination room entering the second time in Cycle 1 and

(Continued next page)

the first time in Cycle 2. The provider will enter the second time in Cycle 2 and the first time in Cycle 3. The staff managing the check-out process can enter the final time in Cycle 3.

Another factor time factor that can be considered in Cycle 1 would be the time that that patient arrives, or checks-in.

The interval times can be calculated by the person responsible for the audit, so as not to delay the patient visit process.

To endeavor to partner with your patients in this improvement effort, you may consider having the patient complete the form during their visit.

MEASURING PATIENT WAITING TIMES:

Cycle 1

Appointment time	
Time patient is escorted to the exam room	
Total elapsed time:	

Cycle 2

Time patient arrives in the exam room	
Time patient is seen by provider	
Total elapsed time	

Cycle 3

Time patient provider visit complete	
Time patient checks-out	
Total elapsed time	

Total door-to-door time: _____

Comments/Observations: _____

_____

_____

_____

Figure 3-4. Wait Time Audit Tool

Other important strategies include making sure patients are greeted with a smile and a warm welcome, no matter how someone feels, and all physicians and advance practice professionals should know the importance of greeting the patient, sitting down eye to eye, asking open-ended questions, not putting the EMR between them and the patient, not using the "busy card" and being aware of and their own body language during the actual visit.

Human Resources. The human resources element of five-star service is critical. Your staff see patients first, last, and cumulatively more often than you do. Therefore, they set the tone for your office and can have a huge impact on your patients' satisfaction levels. Data show that employee satisfaction and patient satisfaction are directly related.

The concept of five-star service should become part of your hiring, orientation, in-service, and employee evaluations. Strive to hire individuals who understand and are committed to your five-star culture. During the orientation process you can further demonstrate the organizational commitment and set expectations. Through educational programs, you will keep the concept in front of your staff. Incorporating five-star service into evaluations shows commitment and can be part of an employee reward system.

The above provides some classic "low-hanging fruit", which you can pick at the start . . . which will provide you with momentum as the early successes are announced.

It is important that you not only provide the tools, but also ensure they are being used appropriately and consistently. This is where your five-star committee can get involved, re-assessing the five-star culture on a regular basis.

Warning: The necessary work of surveying and reducing tolerance for naysayers may create some short-term conflict and stress. However, it may well be exactly what you practice, department, or organization needs.

CHAPTER 4

How to Achieve Internal Five-Star Service

It can be very difficult to create a culture in which your entire organization, whether they are physicians, advanced practice professionals, staff, or management, pervasively and consistently strive for true five-star customer service particularly if they do not *first* exhibit "internal Five five-star" behavior. By this, we mean the way everyone treats each other, particularly in times of stress. We mention stress throughout the book because it is in times of stress that all too often relationships and communications break down. That is when a practice's or organization's five-star culture is challenged. During these times, it is more important than ever to focus on good communication skills, patience, respect, and courtesy. It is about more than keeping one's temper or not being hostile, although both are clearly important. It is also about developing habits to reduce the stress and tension that often exists in an intense work environment.

Internal five-star service deals with how doctors treat each other and the staff, how staff interacts with each other, and how management interacts with physicians, all healthcare professionals, and their staff.

Realistically, you cannot eliminate all stress and tension; therefore, you must learn to manage it. Internal five-star service deals with how doctors treat each other and the staff, how staff interacts with each other, and how management interacts with physicians, all healthcare professionals, and their staff. Of course, it is a two-way street.

You've likely seen how this can play out in a medical practice. If a doctor is chronically late, it causes a backlash with patients because their appointment times are affected. Patients often take a late appointment out on the staff as if it were their fault, and the staff becomes frustrated. The staff may in turn take it out on the doctor. This can anger the doctor because he expects the staff to help with the smooth flow of patients. That one action—being late—begins a vicious cycle of animosity that can intensify throughout the day. When this occurs, it is difficult for the staff to do precisely what the doctor would want under these circumstances: to pour on the five-star service so the patient, who is waiting longer than anticipated, remains calm. This is only one example—there are countless versions of this, but it typically starts with a lack of what we call "internal" five-star service.

Another example involves the impact of life outside of the medical practice. Life can be bumpy at times. Maybe a staff member had a difficult weekend. Perhaps a family member is ill or raising teenage children is proving to be challenging. However, when staff members' frustrations or concerns overflow into the office, patients and staff can see it in body language or verbal cues; it's as if the staff member is saying "stay away from me."

Everyone can sympathize and think of reasons that kind of behavior is understandable. However, in great service-oriented organizations like the Ritz Organization, Disney, and Four Seasons, an individual's frustrations and concerns outside the workplace do not touch the customers. We understand that within the Ritz Organization, there are team meetings in which good managers literally ask employees whether there is anything occurring in their life that could affect their interaction with customers that day. Sometimes concerns are voiced and resolved to the extent possible. It is taken seriously. There must be internal five-star service for true outstanding customer service to take place.

Fortunately, much of these issues can be addressed by training after the staff accepts the true importance of the five-star concept. Physicians, advanced practice professionals, and all employees can be trained around communication issues, strategies to overcome frustration, and body language. Scripts can be created to handle certain circumstances. Some simple strategies that have been used by practices around the country include the following:

Yearly In-Service. Each year, the practice can hold an in-service on service excellence. This is a topic that needs to be front and center each year; it never becomes redundant. The program could incorporate any particular concerns that have arisen during the past year or were brought up in patient experience surveys. Simple to use and pragmatic strategies or tools could be reviewed. The session should be enjoyable, nonjudgmental, and fresh.

We underestimate how powerful recognition can be. Tell someone tomorrow about the good job they have done and they may well pass the good will on.

Recognition. You should recognize employees for service excellence. That recognition could be in the form of an employee of the month with an employee parking spot for that month. The recognition could be published in your newsletter and on your website. Although many will not admit it, recognition for excelling at this important concept is actually important to them. Even just a sincere thank you or observing and pointing out a job well done can go a long way. We underestimate how powerful recognition can be. Tell someone tomorrow about the good job they have done and they may well pass the good will on. Scream at someone in front of patients (yes, this still happens) and imagine the resulting, lingering aftermath.

Annual Employee Opinion Surveys. Taking the pulse of your employees on how they feel about the practice is important. If the questions are specific enough, you can get good information that your five-star committee can use to address concerns. It is important to note that the surveys should not simply be an opportunity for employees to vent or dream—those kinds of responses will not benefit the practice. However, once the five-star culture kicks in, sincere, constructive feedback should be received and can be very useful. See Figure 4-1 for a sample survey.

EMPLOYEE OPINION SURVEY

The survey is ideal for practices with more than ten employees. The Employee Opinion Survey is designed to gather data to be used in improving practice management and operations. Trending answers will assist management in determining where process improvement can be made and where management operations are most effective. Creating a plan of improvement or action based on the outcome data will assist management with operational goal setting for organizational strategic planning.

Feelings about _____ Practice	Strongly Agree	Agree	Disagree	Strongly Disagree
1	If an acquaintance were looking for work, I would recommend_____.				
2	Employee morale is generally good.				
3	_____ provides excellent service/treatment.				
4	Do you understand and work towards meeting _____ mission?				

My Job	Strongly Agree	Agree	Disagree	Strongly Disagree
1	My job is important to _____ success.				
2	The stress of my job is manageable.				
3	I am generally satisfied with my job.				
4	My job description reflects my current job duties/responsibilities.				
5	I understand what is expected of me and I am comfortable being held accountable.				
6	My personal work efforts contribute to the _____ success.				

Quality of Overall Management	Strongly Agree	Agree	Disagree	Strongly Disagree
1	Work rules/policies are equally applied to all employees.				
2	Employee suggestions are encouraged.				
3	I am involved in decision-making that affects my job.				
4	Personnel policies and procedures at _____ are as good or better than at other places where I have worked.				
5	Job assignments are made fairly.				
6	Complaints and problems are handled fairly.				
7	Management runs _____ efficiently and effectively.				
8	When I started working at _____, I was adequately trained to do my job.				
9	Employees are given support and training to improve job performance.				
10	Policies and procedures are enforced equally among departments.				
11	Management has created an open and comfortable work environment.				
12	I am involved in Departmental/Practice training.				

1

Figure 4-1. Sample Employee Opinion Survey, section 1.

New Employee Orientation and Five-Star Attestation. All new employees should receive an orientation to the practice's five-star culture. They must understand the concept generally but also how important service excellence is to your practice and what the expectations are for them. It will be part of their

EMPLOYEE OPINION SURVEY - Section II

Communication	Strongly Agree	Agree	Disagree	Strongly Disagree
1	_____ keeps me informed about things that concern my job and me.			
2	Communication between employees is open and respectful.			
3	I feel free to discuss my problems and/or concerns with my supervisor.			
4	_____ strategic plans are communicated to the staff.			
5	My supervisor communicates policies and procedures to employees.			
6	I have the information I need to do my job properly.			

Working Relationships/Cooperation	Strongly Agree	Agree	Disagree	Strongly Disagree
1	The members in our practice are cooperative.			
2	We work as a team.			
3	I am treated with respect by management and the people I work with.			
4	Management recognizes and makes use of my abilities and skills.			
5	I am encouraged to develop new and more efficient ways to do my work.			
6	The purpose of _____ is clearly identified and understood by employees.			

My Supervisor	Strongly Agree	Agree	Disagree	Strongly Disagree
1	My supervisor knows his/her job well.			
2	Decisions of my supervisor are seldom affected by favoritism.			
3	My supervisor is supportive of me.			
4	My supervisor praises me when I do a good job.			
5	I feel my work is evaluated fairly.			
6	My supervisor communicates current _____ information to me.			
7	My supervisor is open to new ideas.			

Figure 4-1. Sample Employee Opinion Survey, section 2.

evaluations and in part, their compensation calculation. Make it important from the beginning and have the employees sign a short, concise document that attests to the fact that they understand how important five-star service is and that it is part of the practice culture (Figure 3-2). Employees' questions about the value of such a document or concerns about signing it are certainly red flags, but most prospective employees will see it as an example of just how important the concept is and will even see it as a positive reflection of the type of environment in which they want to work.

EMPLOYEE OPINION SURVEY - SECTION III

Pay, Benefits, Upward Mobility	Strongly Agree	Agree	Disagree	Strongly Disagree
1 I am compensated fairly for the job I do.				
2 Pay increases are administered fairly. (Based on job performance, productivity and teamwork)				
3 I understand my benefits plan.				
4 Benefits at _____ are average or better when compared to other places I have worked.				
5 Promotional opportunities at _____ are good compared with other practices our size.				
6 Rank _____ benefits in order of importance to you (1-11):				

    ____Health Insurance   ____Vacation   ____Disability Insurance   ____Holidays
    ____Meals   ____Pension   ____Sick/Personal Time   ____Bereavement Pay
    ____Voluntary Benefits   ____Life Insurance   ____Long-term Disability
    (Dental, Additional Life, Tax-Deferred Annuity)

Safety	Strongly Agree	Agree	Disagree	Strongly Disagree
1 Sufficient attention is given to job safety at _____.				
2 I have received training on Universal Precautions.				
3 I am adequately trained on how to handle a crisis.				
4 I am adequately trained on how to handle disaster situations.				

Comments:

Please state any comments that would help us better understand any survey response that you feel needs clarification.

_____

_____

_____

Figure 4-1. Sample Employee Opinion Survey, section 3.

Five-Star Service Excellence Value Statements. Having a values statement (Figure 3-1)that is kept in front of the employees can help them understand how important this concept is to the practice. Again, your goal is to keep the concept in front of people so it can truly become part of your culture.

A TOTAL COMMITMENT TO INTERNAL FIVE-STAR SERVICE

Five-star service is something that everyone can and should embrace. Physicians can go a long way in creating an internal five-star environment by embracing it themselves and taking it personally. Tasks as simple as starting on time, saying good morning upon reaching the office, sharing a smile, and keeping one's emotions in check are all ways to promote this culture. Physicians are a mirror. Staff will look to them to see if all the talk about five-star service is real or just another passing fad.

Breaches in five-star service should be treated like any other HR issue. If it is at the physician level, it must be addressed by the physician leadership. If it is among the staff, it needs to be handled like any other breach of an important HR policy. Once everyone in the practice has made the commitment and been given the tools, the practice needs to take this issue seriously. Those who need help should receive additional tools; those who simply will not support the program perhaps should not be there.

CHAPTER 5

Moving to External Five-Star Service

The rubber hits the proverbial road with external five-star service. This is where the action is. This is looking at how your patients and their families are treated and feel; it's about *every point of contact* that they have with your office, including:

- How they are treated when they call to schedule an appointment;
- What they see when they log on to your website;
- How they access your patient portal and the interaction;
- How they are treated when they call with an urgent health concern;
- How they are greeted at the reception desk;
- How they are called back (invited) to the exam room;
- The interaction at the actual visit;
- What happens when they have a complaint; and
- How an adverse event is handled.

Not only is it every point of contact, but every member of your office team's interactions with patients as well. Your patients' perceptions of you are affected by how your nurse manages patient care and communication, how your billing personnel respond to patient billing questions, and how your receptionist answers the phone.

Traditionally, healthcare has focused on the *physician*-patient relationship. Of course this is vital to successful outcomes and patient satisfaction; however, an area often neglected by the healthcare industry is the *practice*-patient relationship. As a physician, you could have an excellent relationship with your patients, but if your office is not projecting the same five-star service that you provide, the quality of your patient care and patient satisfaction will diminish.

Let's be clear: Physicians certainly need to be champions and role models. However, excellent service does not stop there. Patients and family members can become frustrated with a practice, and even though they are happy with their doctor, they may not be able to tolerate the office staff and processes. We have heard them say, "I really like Dr. Smith; but I cannot stand his office staff." Yes, many of the patient frustrations stem from changes in healthcare delivery or about their illness or perhaps their health insurer, and you can suffer from the splash-effect However, you can reduce that splash. Data suggest that patients can sort out who is responsible for what. You and your office can be a positive aspect of healthcare changes. We have seen it happen!

Traditionally, healthcare has focused on the *physician*-patient relationship. Of course this is vital to successful outcomes and patient satisfaction; however, an area often neglected by the healthcare industry is the *practice*-patient relationship.

Events that detract from your relationship with the patient can happen and do happen. Realizing they can occur and being pro-active in those areas helps to reduce any potential harm. Let's review a few:

- Inadvertent mistreatment of patients by office staff. Inadvertent because staff do not intend to show disrespect to patients. However, patients pick up on body language, and these days, patient expectations are at an all-time high. Poor body language, an overheard comment taken out of context, lack of eye contact, or signs of being impatient can make a patient feel unwelcomed. Your staff must understand that patients are always listening, always alert to what's going on. Reminding staff that they are always "on" can help to reduce this clearly inadvertent harm.
- Long wait times for appointments. Wait times are of course a long-known patient complaint, that continues. Patients sit in waiting rooms and stew when no one acknowledges that their appointment time has come and gone and no explanation for it is provided to them. The entire situation sets a

negative tone for the staff interaction with the patient and the doctor interaction with the patient. You can be proactive in understanding your patient wait times, and working to reduce wait times. Audit your patient wait time and use the data learned toput into place measures that will help lessen patient anxiety during waits—because you cannot prevent all extended wait times. Place a sign at the registration desk that sets patient expectations and lets them know that their time is valuable to you. For example, post a sign such as: "We are sorry if you are waiting longer than anticipated. We respect your time. If you are 15 minutes past your appointment time, please see the receptionist." We have seen this strategy work effectively.

Technology can also help physician practices with this common complaint. Smartphone and tablet apps are being created that will help practices keep patients informed of delays. Further, one new patient engagement app will provide greater efficiencies to practices by permitting patients to complete paper work and medical issue documentation in advance of the visit. Further, make sure that valuable educational materials are available in reception areas.

- Scheduling: Long wait times for physician appointments. Some patients prefer to see a physician rather than a PA, and are not happy when told that the doctor is not available for an appointment for another two weeks or more. With the increased number of insureds and the resultant increased demand on the physician practices, combined with the need to incorporate advanced healthcare practice professionals into the day-to-day patient care at physician practices, this is becoming more of a hot topic in the industry. Patients who want to see a physician, but simply cannot wait the length of time it would take to get an appointment with the physician, can become irritated and angry. Information in the next chapter can help physicians address this area, as patient engagement becomes a key concept in patient care and advanced practice professionals are recognized as part of the patient's care team.

- Patients seeing or hearing staff or physicians arguing with each other. We underestimate how unsettling this is to patients. It is natural that professionals will disagree and there are settings where it is appropriate to do so (QA, peer review for example). However, when it takes place in a public setting, patients or their families can misinterpret what they are seeing or hearing. Did someone do something wrong? Why is the doctor so upset? Is he distracted? Angry words between doctors or staff are never viewed as a positive by a patient or family and they are never forgotten.

Five-star service has always been important, but has become even more so now that national healthcare reform will affect the way healthcare is delivered in this country and how practices are reimbursed for the care provided. Reimbursement is moving from volume-based to value-based reimbursement. Measurement of value will include the patient experience ratings. So now, patient satisfaction is not just about maintaining a good physician-patient relationship, it can also affect your finances.

> **Five-star service has always been important, but has become even more so now that national healthcare reform will affect the way healthcare is delivered in this country and how practices are reimbursed for the care provided.**

More specifically, an Accountable Care Organization, in order to participate in shared savings, must meet quality standards for a given year, and 7 of the 33 standards are related to "patient care giver experience." These 7 measures are captured from CAHPS surveys.[1]

The concept of the patient experience is one that began to take hold in the healthcare industry only recently. For example, the Cleveland Clinic created the Office of Patient Experience, designed to address every aspect of patient care, including emotional well-being, comfort, and education. This includes healthcare giver interactions, patient and caregiver interactions, communication, cleanliness, healing initiatives, and noise levels during evening hours, just to name a few.[2]

External five-star service is critically important, particularly with the future transparency regarding patient satisfaction. However, these are all building blocks: having internal five-star service in place, having a plan, getting the training to start you successfully in this path. Now let's discuss staying there.

References

1. Patient Protection and Affordable Care Act of 2010, Pub. L. No. 111-148, sec 3022 124 (2010); Medicare Program; Medicare Shared Savings Program: Accountable Care Organizations, 76 FR 67801, Issue 212 (Nov. 2, 2011).

2. For more information, see: http://my.clevelandclinic.org/patient_experience/default.aspx.

CHAPTER 6

Post-Adverse Event
Communication and
Disclosure

P ost-adverse event communication and disclosure are important parts of a
patient-centric environment, While becoming more accepted concepts,
some confusion remains among doctors, lawyers, and even patients.

Let's first get a basic understanding of post-adverse event communication.
It is just what it sounds like: verbal communication that a physician or other
healthcare professionals have with a patient and/or a patient's family *after* a
patient suffers an adverse outcome, regardless of whether the outcome is a known
complication or an actual error that occurred during the course of medical care.

Doctors are often concerned that he will be perceived by patients and/
or families as accepting responsibility (fault) for an adverse outcome during
this post-adverse event communication, thereby exposing the doctor or other
healthcare professionals or an entity to liability. This is a valid concern; certainly
there are instances when patients or their families misconstrued a doctor's discussion about an adverse event or words of empathy as an admission of fault or
negligence. It is true that what is said after an adverse event occurs and how it
is said can affect liability risk and a patient's decision to see a lawyer. Witman
and colleagues concluded that patients are more likely to sue when a physician
does not disclose an error;[1] however, post-adverse event communications, when
stated in the right context, at the right time, with the right preparation, can help
reduce liability exposure, and is clearly the right approach for the patient and
the doctor.

Context is the key. For example, by simply stating, "I'm sorry," a doctor is leaving it up to the patient to fill in the blanks. The doctor says "I'm sorry," but the patient hears: "I'm sorry for cutting your common bile duct," or "I'm sorry; your injury is all my fault."

The key is not giving the patient an opportunity to fill in any blanks. An appropriate statement showing empathy but not admitting liability can look like:

> "We have determined the cause of your mother's leg pain to be a blood clot. This is a potential complication of any knee surgery, and I had discussed that with your mother when we talked about this surgery. I am saddened that she has this additional condition to deal with during her recovery, but know that a treatment plan is underway and we will continue to monitor the clot."

Many states have enacted laws to encourage open dialogue between patients and their healthcare providers in these instances—they are often called "apology laws" but you might also hear them called "sorry laws," "immunity laws," or "empathy laws." According to the American Medical Association, 37 states had some form of an apology law in 2012 (see http://www.ama-assn.org/resources/doc/arc/apology-inadmissibility-state-laws-charts.pdf). In October 2013, Pennsylvania brought the number to 38, when Pennsylvania Governor Tom Corbett signed S.B. 379, permitting healthcare providers to express a "benevolent gesture" without it being used against them in the courtroom (under certain circumstances).[2] If your state has one of these laws, it is important to know it and understand it: What's protected? What's not? Who is protected? Who is not protected?

This is why many institutions educate their healthcare professionals about disclosure and communication issues. While these laws intend to foster open communication and simultaneously reduce liability risk, if the communication is not done within the bounds of the legislation, or is not done effectively, it has the potential of negatively affecting liability risk for physicians and healthcare providers. The complete opposite effect intended.

The education and training necessary is not difficult and clearly is a worthwhile endeavor. The educational endeavor should be coordinated and incorporate all the stakeholders from the beginning: physicians, nurses, staff, hospital leadership, risk management, defense counsel, and claims management. Elements of the training may include the following:

- Education for the entire practice about what post-adverse event communication is and the organizational commitment to it. An outside speaker or speakers can be hired to provide different perspectives; often times it is more effective for physicians to hear from physicians and defense counsel to hear from defense counsel.
- Training for the post-adverse event communicators: physicians, leadership, clergy, and others. This is the literal "how to" with role playing, examples, and resources.
- Finally, "train the trainers" for sustainability of your culture.

The apology laws can help to align the relevant post-adverse event communication players: Patients, doctors, risk managers, defense lawyers, and medical professional liability insurers and be an impetus for the education.

The apology laws can help to align the relevant post-adverse event communication players: Patients, doctors, risk managers, defense lawyers, and medical professional liability insurers and be an impetus for the education.

Now, with an understanding of what post-adverse event communication is, you need to have the opportunity to communicate with a patient and family after an adverse event occurs. Enhancing your chances of having that opportunity requires preparation long before the event ever actually happens. Let's review the concept of five-star service excellence as the mechanism that allows you to transcend the event.

WHEN AN ADVERSE EVENT HAPPENS

Five-star culture allows physicians and patients to develop a trusting relationship that will transcend an adverse event. Having this in place from the start enhances the chances that when an adverse outcome occurs, patients will return to their doctors for the discussion and be prepared to truly listen to what their doctors have to say. Patients and their families will have questions, and you do not want them trying to get answers to them on their own, with input from friends or a plaintiff's lawyer. They should look to you for information first.

Effective post-adverse event communication is not a moment in time; it is connected to a continuum that begins with five-star service (Figure 6-1).

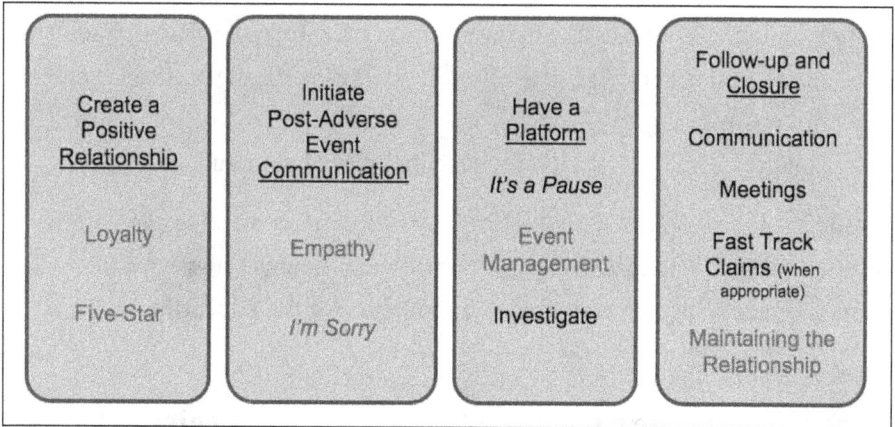

Create a Positive Relationship	Initiate Post-Adverse Event Communication	Have a Platform	Follow-up and Closure
Loyalty	Empathy	It's a Pause	Communication
Five-Star	I'm Sorry	Event Management	Meetings
		Investigate	Fast Track Claims (when appropriate)
			Maintaining the Relationship

Figure 6-1. Continuum of Effective Communication

Loyal patients are the key to transcending an event. How do you know that you have a loyal patient population? In part, you know based on the answer to that specialty-specific survey question, "How likely are you (patient) to return to this practice?" or "How likely are you to refer this practice to a family member or friend?" or a similarly phrased question. The answer is a strong predictor of satisfaction and loyalty. It also is part of the CAHPS surveying discussed earlier in this book and the specialty-specific survey distributed by MedStatix that we discussed in Chapter 2. It all circles back to knowing and understanding your patients' wants, desires, and needs, and delivering on them.

Establishing the loyal, trusting patient relationship begins with the first contact a patient has with a practice. It is the age-old "first impression," which can be a lasting impression. This fact supports the recommendation that five-star service must be a pervasive culture within your organization, because you never know what impression is going to be created at any given time, at any part of the patient's exposure to your practice.

For healthcare professionals who provide surgical services, the informed consent form can be helpful in setting patient expectations from the beginning, that you will be available to speak with them, and want to speak with them, if the surgical procedure results are not as planned. In the consent form, you can literally let your patients know that if there is an adverse outcome, you, the physician, are available to the patient and family to discuss the matter and answer their questions. Many practices around the country have incorporated the following paragraph onto their informed consent form:

> "In the unlikely event that one or more of the above complications may occur, my doctor will take appropriate and reasonable steps to help manage the clinical situation and be available to me and my family to address our concerns and questions."

SO, WHAT DO YOU DO WHEN AN ADVERSE EVENT OCCURS?

With the stage set with a solid physician-patient relationship, to transcend an event, what should you do when the event happens? Many times in the past, physicians would want to talk with their patients but were reluctant to do so because of liability concerns, and some are actually discouraged. Again, here is when the state "apology laws" can support post-adverse event communication.

First and foremost, always, always, always empathize with your patient and the patient's family.

First and foremost, always, always, always empathize with your patient and the patient's family. No matter who you are or what happened, empathy is always appropriate. It should be heartfelt and sincere (patients know when it is not). Empathy is also desired by patients and well-received when sincere.

What you do next depends on the type of adverse event that occurred. Adverse events can be categorized as follows:

1. A known complication or risk of a procedure or treatment plan;
2. An actual medical error, generally described as a preventable adverse outcome; or
3. Neither (possibly a service issue).

Why are these distinctions important? Determining if the adverse event is a complication of a surgical or medical procedure or a true medical error influences your communication. Adverse/negative outcomes make up 100% of medical malpractice claims. That is, you cannot have a medical malpractice claim without an injury to redress. Certainly not every adverse outcome is the result of medical malpractice. A known complication or risk of a procedure or treatment plan is not medical malpractice; actual medical error (a preventable adverse outcome) could be.

Determining what type of adverse event occurred may require an investigation (done in an appropriate and often confidential fashion), an RCA, discussion with hospital risk management, and/or discussion with your medical professional liability insurer.

Now, let's look at how to respond to each scenario.

1. An investigation reveals the adverse event was a known potential complication.

This will be the majority of events. In addition to empathy, provide information about what happened using known, objective facts. Do not guess or speculate about what occurred; if you don't know, say so, but follow up. Discuss what is being done to reduce any further harm or injury. Again, if you are not clear about what caused the injury at this time, say so, then answer any questions the patient may have. Provide the patient with your contact information for any future questions.

If your informed consent form included the statement noted above, reference that document and its contents and your discussion if necessary:

> "Remember during our discussion about the surgery to remove your gallbladder we talked about the known risks associated with this surgery? Particularly I had pointed out the risk of a transected bile duct. During your procedure, this did occur. It was immediately recognized and repaired. I inserted a drain that is needed and will be there temporarily. We will schedule a time to have it removed. I'm going to have you stay in the hospital for continued observation, because the drain is in place. Of course, we feel terrible and I am so sorry this occurred..."
> (Figure 6-2 is a Third Generation Informed Consent Form.)

Key takeaways:
- **Always express empathy**
- **Put "I'm sorry" into context.**

INFORMED CONSENT FOR CHOLECYSTECTOMY

It is very important to [insert physician, practice name] that you understand and consent to the treatment your doctor is providing for you and any procedure your doctor may perform. You should be involved in any and all decisions concerning surgical procedures your doctor has recommended. Sign this form only after you understand the procedure, the anticipated benefits, the risks, the alternatives, the risks associated with the alternatives and all of your questions have been answered. Please initial and date directly below this paragraph indicating your understanding of this paragraph.

_____   _____

Patient's Initials or Authorized Representative   Date

I, _____, hereby authorize Dr._____ and any associates or assistants the doctor deems appropriate, to perform an open cholecystectomy.

This procedure involves the surgical removal of the gallbladder, an organ located just under the liver on the upper right of the abdomen. The gallbladder stores and concentrates bile, a substance produced by the liver. In the open method of surgery, a two to --three inch incision is made on the right upper side of the abdomen. The surgeon locates the gallbladder and removes it through the incision.

The doctor has explained the benefits of the procedure(s) to me. However, I understand there is no certainty that I will achieve these benefits and no guarantee has been made to me regarding the outcome of the procedure(s). I also authorize the administration of sedation and/or anesthesia as may be deemed advisable or necessary for my comfort, well-being and safety.

Risks: The doctor has explained to me that there are risks and possible undesirable consequences associated with this procedure that may occur during my surgery or during my recuperation *including, but not limited to*: bleeding, infection, injury to the bile duct (the tube that carries bile from the gallbladder to the small intestine), bile leak, blood clots, heart problems such as cardiac arrhythmias or heart attack, damage to the pancreas, pancreatitis and/or death injury.

I understand that if I need blood or blood products these carry a risk of contracting HIV/AIDS, hepatitis, or other diseases.

In permitting my doctor to perform the procedure(s), I understand that unforeseen conditions may be revealed that may necessitate change or extension of the original procedure(s) or a different procedure(s) than those already explained to me. I therefore authorize and request that the above-named physician, his assistants, or his designees perform such procedure(s) as necessary and desirable in the exercise of his/her professional judgment.

In the unlikely event that one or more of the above complications occur, my physician(s) will take appropriate and reasonable steps to help manage the clinical situation and be available to me and my family to address our concerns and questions.

Figure 6-2. Third Generation Informed Consent Form (page 1).

2. An investigation reveals the adverse event was a medical error.

The same advice about what to do when a known potential complication occurs applies here as well: empathize; provide objective, known facts; discuss what happened; and discuss what is being done further to reduce any harm. However,

Alternatives to the Procedure: The reasonable alternative(s) to the procedure(s) have been explained to me. These alternatives *include, but are not limited to*: watchful waiting, increased exercise, diet changes, laparoscopic transcystic common bile duct stone extraction or ERCP.

Risks to Alternatives: I understand the risks associated with the alternatives *include, but are not limited to*: worsening of symptoms, infection, pancreatitis, perforation of adjacent organs, bleeding or bursting of the gallbladder

I hereby authorize the doctor to utilize or dispose of removed tissues, parts or organs resulting from the procedure(s) authorized above.

I consent to any photographing or videotaping of the procedure(s) that may be performed, provided my identity is not revealed by the pictures or by descriptive texts accompanying them. I consent to the admittance of students or authorized equipment representatives to the procedure room for purposes of advancing medical education or obtaining important product information.

By signing below, I certify that I have had an opportunity to ask the doctor all my questions concerning anticipated benefits, material risks, alternatives, and risks of those alternatives, and all of my questions have been answered to my satisfaction.

_____/_____/_____   _____
Date   Time   Signature of Patient or Authorized Representative   Relationship of Authorized Representative

❑   The Patient/Authorized Representative has read this form or had it read to him/her.

❑   The Patient/Authorized Representative states that he/she understands this information.

❑   The Patient/Authorized Representative has no further questions.

_____   _____   _____
Date   Time   Signature of Witness

CERTIFICATION OF PHYSICIAN:

I hereby certify that I have discussed with the individual granting consent, the facts, anticipated benefits, material risks, alternative therapies and the risks associated with the alternatives of the procedure(s).

_____   _____   _____
Date   Time   Signature of Physician

USE OF INTERPRETER OR SPECIAL ASSISTANCE

An interpreter or special assistance was used to assist patient in completing this form as follows:

_____Foreign language (specify)

Figure 6-2. Third Generation Informed Consent Form (page 2).

in these situations, it is also important to accept responsibility, *if a due diligence investigation results in an opinion that an error occurred and that error resulted in an injury to the patient.*

_____Sign language

_____Patient is blind, form read to patient

_____Other (specify)_____

Interpretation provided by _____

(Fill in name of Interpreter and Title or Relationship to Patient)

_____   _____   _____
Signature (Individual Providing Assistance)   Date   Time

Figure 6-2. Third Generation Informed Consent Form (page 3).

By due diligence, we mean an appropriate level of investigation into the facts and circumstances. Sometimes this will require a review of the matter by a clinical expert. Through the review you can get an understanding of standard of care issues and causation (both elements to proving negligence). It will aid in discussions with the patient and/or family, who may be skeptical about the conclusions reached and which may be seen otherwise as self-serving.

Some investigations will take longer than others. The key is to assure patient safety first and keep the patient/family informed of what you are doing so they do not think that nothing is happening and you have "blown them off." Depending on the circumstances, investigations can include a physician, a subsequent physician, a nurse, a hospital risk manager, a hospital's lawyer, the physicians' lawyers, and the insurance carriers for the doctors for example, and this is why a considerable amount of time can lapse.

Further, be aware of discovery and confidentiality issues. If you follow a confidential process, you are more apt to receive cooperation from your staff, which will help get to the real facts and circumstances. In addition, a confidential process can prevent the leak of information too early or unconfirmed information that would have a negative impact on the post-adverse event communication. Control the investigation and the flow of information. There is no nefarious intention here, simply a matter of appropriate process for optimal results for everyone.

The review should determine whether the standard of care was breached and whether that the breach was the cause of the patient's injury. It's possible that a medication error occurred, but that error did not cause an injury to the patient. This is a difficult conversation to have with a patient and/or family member because you need to explain that you did something wrong, but that it did not cause the injury that the patient sustained. Certainly that is good news to the patient, but you would be surprised how difficult these conversations can be. This is why involving your medical professional liability insurance lawyer in preparing for patient/family discussions and meetings can be beneficial.

Research by Gallagher, et al. sets forth patient desires when it comes to "disclosing an error."[3] Patients want:

1. Disclosure of the error;
2. To understand what happened;
3. To understand why the error happened;
4. To know how the consequences of the error will be mitigated;
5. To be assured recurrences will be prevented; and
6. Emotional support, including an apology (acceptance of responsibility, when appropriate).

The Institute of Medicine Report (1999) concluded that most medical errors are the result of systems errors. Some examples to consider include:

- Vicryl sutures used on a patient where the patient had an allergy to the sutures as documented in the office chart, but not part of the hospital chart. At the hospital, the surgical tray was prepared by a hospital nurse. Although you performed the surgery, one of your assistant surgeons actually closed the patient. The patient could initially blame you. But, there is a system issue here involving transfer of information between the office and hospital.
- You prescribed Lasix for a patient, however, a miscommunication occurred between your nurse and office secretary resulted in the patient being given a script for Toperal 20 mg. The pharmacy called your office because Toperal does not come in 20 mg. Your receptionist said to go ahead and give the patient the 25 mg daily dosage. This is a system issue—your receptionist should not be providing medical advice.

When these types of events occur, let the patient know what is being done to prevent the same from occurring to anyone else in the future.

An example of an appropriate communication after a medical error is determined from due diligence:

"You received 2 times the dose of medicine than was intended. We do not yet understand why that occurred, but are investigating to determine why it did. Once we have more information, we will discuss that with you further. In the meantime, please know that your laboratory tests and vital signs are being closely monitored. We do not anticipate any harmful impact to you. We cannot tell you how sorry we are that this occurred."

Key takeaways:
- **Accept responsibility when due diligence has determined it to be appropriate.**
- **Coordinate with your legal counsel before accepting responsibility.**
- **Prepare. (More on this later.)**

3. *What if there is no actual adverse event but a patient perceives that an adverse event occurred?*

A service lapse should also be addressed, but addressed differently than a complication or true medical error. This is a key point. Practices often ignore a service lapse as just one of those unfortunate events that occurs; however, the service lapse is one of the types of aggravating factors that actually prompts patients to see a lawyer when an adverse event does occur. It may not be that an adverse event is associated with this particular service lapse, but if an adverse event happens later, and the patient recalls that the service issue was never handled, the patient's frustrations continue to linger and perhaps even build. The patient is now more likely to become upset or frustrated by the event and may even seek a lawyer rather than returning to talk to you. These aggravating circumstances also are often what make cases attractive to a plaintiff's lawyer, as they can be used to inflame a jury and increase the value of a settlement or jury award. So, the service lapses must not be ignored.

What happens at your practice when a patient makes a complaint? Do you know? The reality is that most complaints could have a germ of truth associated with them, and they are opportunities to set your five-star service platform into motion. They are also learning opportunities to prevent similar complaints in the future.

The type of complaint whereby a patient perceives inappropriate care or treatment, when in fact the care was appropriate, can also fall under this category. Failing to address these types of matters can result in a lawsuit, which will take time to get dismissed.

The matter may not appear important to you, but it is important to the patient. When patients do not get an attorney to take on a case for them, they have an alternative means of pursuing a resolution: they can file a complaint with your state medical board. We have seen an uptick in the number of complaints lodged against physicians to state medical boards. The complaint is likely the result of consolidation of plaintiff counsel and the lack of monetary value in certain allegations; however, every state medical board takes *every* patient complaint seriously and investigates each one. Defending yourself in one of these state board matters can be time consuming. The best defense is a great offense. In other words, deal with the patient complaints and service issues when they occur; it could go a long way in preventing further headaches for you with the state medical board and associated implications.

State medical boards may have a different standard of review than a standard negligence lawsuit (it may be a lesser burden); and adverse actions against you by a state board can result in additional adverse impacts. For example, health insurers may remove you from their plans. Other states where you have a license may initiate action based on the outcome of the first state or suspend your license or set a financial penalty. Again, the key is to prevent a state board complaint in the first place. But if one is made, take it seriously. Notify your medical professional liability carrier who may provide you with some partial insurance coverage or reimbursement to manage a response to a state board complaint.

Key takeaway:
Invest in managing service issues when they occur; not only can you prevent a lawsuit or state board complaint, you can also strengthen the physician-patient relationship

What Not To Do After an Adverse Event

There is a tendency at times to try to shift blame to another provider or a nurse, for example. Don't! Doing so just aggravates the situation. Allow the investigation and analysis to take place. Responsibility will fall in the appropriate places.

Examples of post-adverse event communication *to avoid* include:

"Well, if I had known then, what I know now, I would not have recommended the surgery."

"I cut your common bile duct during surgery. I have done this surgery thousands of times and this is the only time in my career it has happened. I just do not know how I did this; it was a mistake."

"I really thought that your mother was a good candidate for bariatric surgery. Now I can see that she probably wasn't. I wish I hadn't told her to have this procedure."

"This shouldn't have happened. We see it happen every few hundred births. I wish I could have prevented it. Your baby will now need to be seen by a pediatrician and we will not know whether he will recover use of his arm for quite some time."

There is a tendency at times to try to shift blame to another provider or a nurse, for example. Don't! Doing so just aggravates the situation. Allow the investigation and analysis to take place. Responsibility will fall in the appropriate places.

Some Tips for Communication Regardless of the Type of Adverse Event

Physicians can be hard on themselves, taking responsibility when they are not responsible. They may also use the "retroscope" to determine that in hindsight, they should have done something differently. Analyze situations based on the -known information at the time the decision was made, without the retroscope, and include your risk management or legal counsel in evaluating the circumstances using an objective process.

Here are 10 key communication tips:

1. Provide patients with a number where you can be reached if there are additional questions.
2. Remember your body language—*you are being watched closely!*
3. Consider confidentiality. Make sure your discussions cannot be heard by those who should not hear them.
4. Make sure you can have your conversation with your patients without being interrupted; show them this respect.
5. Give patients an opportunity to express their thoughts and ask questions.
6. Really listen.

7. Be compassionate and understanding of perspectives—not defensive.
8. Turn off your phone and your beeper.
9. Consider whether you should have another healthcare provider with you as a witness.
10. Consider whether you should follow up with a letter to the patient? Should you document the meeting in the medical chart? And if so, what should it say?

AFTER THE COMMUNICATION—WHAT'S NEXT?

After disclosure, remember that it may not mean that "it's over." Recall the continuum mentioned at the beginning of this chapter. Communication with the patient/family may need to continue. The type of communication depends on the type of event as well as the nature of the event. Each event needs to be handled in a customized fashion. There may be a need for additional meetings or phone calls. There may be a need for a follow-up letter. Whatever the next steps are, remember that there does need to be a balance—if you are too aggressive in trying to communicate with the patient or family, they may get the wrong idea. The goal is that the patient feels supported and that the questions he or she has are answered.

In some cases, when an error has occurred, there may also be the need to make the patient/family whole in some way. With medical errors, that resolution is most often through a payment, but not always. Recall the desire of patients to know that the same event will not happen again to someone else. Often times this can be the basis for a resolution of a situation. For example, it may be a commitment by a hospital for the obstetrical nursing staff to undergo formalized education and training on electronic fetal heart monitoring or a commitment by a doctor to change a process or procedure. Whatever the resolution, most times you will also want to get a "release," document signed by the patient which is yet another reason to involve your medical professional liability defense lawyer. The contents of and when to use a release are outside the scope of this book, but it is important that you understand the general concept that a release documents the completion of a transaction that resolves any complaints or potential complaints that the patient has related to a specific adverse event, and signs off that they understand that and cannot bring a claim against you at a later time involving the immediate circumstance.

There is little doubt that meetings with the patient and/or family will be needed. When they are, take them seriously, and prepare. Collaborate with other healthcare providers, risk management, and legal counsel, as needed. Determine:

- Who will be at the meeting?
- Who will speak at the meeting? What will they say?
- Where will the meeting be held?
- How much time do you have?
- Are there special needs of the patient or family member that need to be addressed for the meeting?

It is an investment of time for sure, but well worth it in preventing three to five years of litigation.

Next Steps

When you know liability exists and a suit will be filed, consider "fast tracking" the claim. Rather than enduring the litigation process and expense, only to end up at the same point where liability is determined, negotiate a pre-suit settlement. Obtain a release as above. Of course, this should be done in collaboration with your medical malpractice insurance carrier and defense attorney.

Additionally, after an event has been handled, use your adverse events as a quality improvement opportunity. Look at both the clinical issues and the professional liability issues. You may determine there is a need to address an opportunity directly with a clinician involved in the patient's care; or you may find that a system issue needs to be addressed. The key is to use the information to enhance quality of care and prevent future similar instances.

A side note: A majority of states require written notification to patients when "serious events" or the like occur. The responsibility for notification often lies with a hospital or ambulatory surgery center. If done well and appropriately, this notification can enhance the loyal relationship; if not done well, it could lead patients directly to a lawyer.

Patient notification of a serious event needs to be a *process*—one that involves all stakeholders working collaboratively (physician and hospital for example), and includes not only a written notification that most states require, but also a conversation between the patient and the healthcare professional. That conversation may be in addition to the post-adverse event communication discussed previously.

It is in the best interest of the hospital and the physician for there to be a collaborative process. Often times, hospitals will discuss the matter with the doctor and allow him to see a copy of the draft letter going to the patient before it is finalized, and soliciting some input. Physicians should ensure the letter is accurate and provides context for the event. Such a process can be helpful in preventing patient misperceptions about the incident, assuming negligence occurred when none may have occurred.

Don't Forget the Patient's Family

This is a good time to further emphasize the role of a patient's family in five-star service and post-adverse event communication. Throughout this book, we mention the patient and *family* multiple times. Involving family in post-event discussions is a new area of emphasis. Even though a patient may have been well-prepared for certain care or a procedure and understand the risks, family members may be unaware. When a patient experiences a significant complication and is not able to communicate (or even dies), it will typically be a family member that becomes responsible for or push for a lawsuit. Setting family members' expectations from the outset, just as you do with the patient, can be important, particularly in higher-risk specialties like obstetrics. You should include the family members in discussions after an event has occurred regardless of prior communications, although, of course, any discussions with family must be consistent with confidentiality and privacy laws.

The Importance of Post-adverse Event Communication for You

For the individual physician(s) and medical practice, you can personally benefit from the concepts outlined in this chapter: closure early for you, closure early for your patient, an enhanced practice environment, enhanced patient satisfaction, and enhanced employee satisfaction. Emotionally it is often what doctors want to do, and it is an added benefit that, when done correctly, can negate or minimize the liability concerns.

We need to move to a culture whereby the doctor-patient relationship truly transcends the adverse event. The doctor and patient (and family) work through concerns, fears, and questions together. There is now an abundance of data that this is truly in the best interest of the patient as well as the physician and hospital.

Additional Benefits of Proper Post-Adverse Event Communication

Above we explained the benefits of a five-star culture as a foundation to effective post-adverse event communication. No discussion of post-adverse event communication would be complete without also identifying the multitude of benefits associated with it. They include decreased lawsuits, reduced payments to settle claims or awarded on claims, and reduced expenses associated with litigation[4]

WHAT SHOULD YOU DO NEXT?

First, your platforms must be in place: your five-star service culture and your culture of safety. These provide the foundation for your post-adverse event communication. So, evaluate your culture of safety and five-star service culture to assure the appropriate climate for the post-adverse event communication concept can take hold. Otherwise your efforts will be fruitless. This evaluation could include:

- An objective, third-party evaluation of the culture of safety;
- Use of the AHRQ culture of safety perception survey; and
- A five-star service evaluation.

Assure as well that a policy and procedure, vetted, is in place concerning the management of medical errors. This provides a structure for when an adverse event does occur. Educate all staff on the policy and procedure. The concept should be a system-wide, practice-wide concept.

References

1. Witman AB, Park DM, Hardin SB. "How do patients want physicians to handle mistakes? A survey of internal medicine patients in an academic setting." *Arch Intern Med.* 1996; 156:2565–2569.

2. See Pennsylvania's Benevolent Gesture Medical Professional Liability Act, Act of Oct. 25, 2013, P.L. 665, No. 79 (2013).

3. Gallagher TH, Waterman AD, Ebers AG, Fraser VJ, and Levinson W. "Patients and physicians' attitudes regarding the disclosure of medical errors." *JAMA.* 2003; 289:1001-1007.

4. See, e.g., Kachalia A, Kaufman SR, Boothman R, et al. "Liability claims and costs before and after implementation of a medical error disclosure program." *Annals of Internal Medicine.* 17 August 2010, 153:4.

CHAPTER 7

Moving from Patient Experience to True Patient Engagement

P ractices that are ahead of the curve on the patient experience are moving closer to true patient engagement. Data show that true patient engagement is one of the keys to enhancing patient adherence to care plans as well as outcomes. Patient engagement also has significant liability mitigation implications. However, the actual implementation of true patient engagement in the physician office can be difficult. It requires changing the way medicine has traditionally been delivered. While any change can be difficult, change in systems and processes during a time of unprecedented change in the healthcare industry can seem like an insurmountable task.

Health Policy Expert: Diane Pinakiewicz, MBA, CPPS

To learn more about the concept of patient engagement, the authors interviewed Diane Pinakiewicz, MBA, CPPS, immediate past president of The National Patient Safety Foundation (2003-2012), and named one of 50 Experts Leading the Field of Patient Safety by *Becker's Hospital Review* (2013). Ms. Pinakiewicz has spent many years evaluating and understanding patient engagement and its role in patient safety, and has specific experiences in various aspects of the healthcare industry, including as an executive at Memorial Sloan Kettering Cancer Center; a senior hospital-based executive for the Hospital Corporation of America, UMDNJ University Hospital; a chief administrative and financial officer at Corning Franklin Health, Inc., a senior director of the Health Care Strategic Leadership Unit at Schering-Plough Pharmaceuticals;

and the vice president of managed care programs at The Brooklyn Hospital Center.

Q1: How is "patient engagement" different from the concept of "patient experience," and how are they alike?

Patient engagement and patient experience are related, yet distinct components of patient-centered care. Patient engagement can be defined as meaningful, informed collaboration between providers and patients to achieve mutually agreed-upon healthcare goals. It requires an informed and activated patient, desirous of assuming a role in his or her health and healthcare, and informed providers who support and welcome the patient onto the healthcare team. This is very different from the traditional patient/provider relationship where the patient has been more passive and the care team, defined without the patient, has created care plans and made critical decisions with little input from the patient. The provider focus has been on the clinical condition of the patient, where the provider expertise lies. Consideration of patient concerns, preferences, values, and the patient's ability to understand and follow the care plan have not been a priority nor have clinicians been trained to solicit and respond to this type of information.

Practices that are ahead of the curve on the patient experience are moving closer to true patient engagement.

Patients, on the other hand, are no longer willing to have little or no voice in their care and want to be informed and involved in matters related to their health, in ways that work for them. They do not want to be defined solely by their clinical conditions but rather respected as human beings who have a right to be fully informed and engaged in their own healthcare. In order to engage, patients must be activated, willing, and able to take action necessary to manage their healthcare to goals. This often requires new skills as well as an ability to seek out and utilize information necessary to allow for informed participation in the care process.

For true patient engagement to occur, patients and providers alike must develop new skill sets and change the ways they behave and the ways they relate to each other. Patients must become informed, willing to take responsibility, and willing and able to speak up for themselves. Providers must be receptive to this, willing to listen and answer questions, able to communicate effectively, and committed to involving the patient in decisions about that patient's care — decisions that respect and incorporate patient point of view, preference, and values. Improving the dynamics of the healing relationship through improved patient engagement is important for all involved and brings value to all in terms of better patient experience, greater provider satisfaction and, as is just beginning to be understood, better clinical and financial outcomes.

To be able to do this, individuals must have sufficient and appropriate information that they can understand and that allows them to be effective members of their own healthcare teams and participants in decisions that affect their well-being.

Patient experience of care defines how a *patient perceives* the care process as performing against criteria that the patient values and holds important. The Beryl Institute describes it as "the sum of all interactions, shaped by an organization's culture, that influence patient perception across the continuum of care." It is important to understand that patient experience of care is described from the patient viewpoint and defined by what matters to the patient. It is not the same as the traditional concept of patient satisfaction, which was a measure of how well providers met the needs of the patient, as providers understood and defined those needs.

Patient experience of care is based on the patient's definition of what is important. This deeper understanding of what matters most to patients has been arrived at through extensive research funded by AHRQ and is reflected in the CAHPS survey instruments. We now understand that, to provide the patient with a good care experience, it is important to communicate frequently and effectively with them, to manage their pain, to ensure that their medications are reconciled— things more meaningful than amenities like valet parking and food choices. While the work in this area is relatively new, improving the patient experience of care comprises one of the three components of the triple aim for improving the healthcare system, the other two being improvement in the overall health of the population and the reduction of healthcare costs.

Patient engagement, when effectively practiced by both the patient and provider, can contribute positively to the patient experience and, together, these two concepts represent elements of the customer focus in healthcare known as patient-centeredness.

Q2: Why is the concept of "patient engagement" so important in today's healthcare environment (to patients and healthcare professionals)?

Effective patient engagement has many potential benefits for patients and healthcare professionals. From the patient perspective, it allows for a level of involvement in one's own healthcare that is being sought by today's consumer. If working correctly within the context of a good relationship/good care team, it facilitates the patient's ability to ask questions, state preferences, make informed choices, raise concerns, follow care plans, help protect against unsafe practices, and ensure responsiveness to things that matter to the patient.

For providers, patient engagement also has a variety of benefits. It provides a means for enriching the provider-patient relationship by aligning the parties around mutually agreed-upon goals for the patient's health and the care plans to achieve those goals. Engaged patients assume responsibilities as part of the care team and can better support, and therefore optimize, their care plans, a key goal of the provider. Providers report higher levels of job satisfaction when they are working with patients in this manner. Providers who engage effectively with their patients and whose patients have better experiences can expect to be better positioned to attract and retain a patient base, particularly as the system becomes more transparent and patients consider this aspect of provider performance as they make their healthcare choices.

Patient engagement is also important to physicians because of its associated financial implications. Some of these relate to optimizing payment and some to minimizing malpractice exposure and expense. With regard to payment, patient experience of care, which is positively influenced by patient engagement, is factoring into every aspect of payment reform. Volume-driven, fee-for-service payment is being replaced with payment based on value delivered, and that value is being defined around quality and safety, reasonableness of cost, and patient experience of care. Value-based purchasing, value-based modifiers for physician payment, PQRS measures, meaningful use requirements for EHR deployment, CAHPS measures, potential modifications to the SGR system, patient-centered medical home and specialty practice recognition programs all factor in standards and incentives related to patient experience and all are influencing payment to physicians. There are incentives for performing well on patient experience of care and penalties for not, and this focus will increase as the system continues to reshape.

In addition to directly affecting a physician's reimbursement, performance with regard to patient engagement will be a factor as partnering decisions are made. As the system moves to new payment models where clinical and financial responsibility for patients are assumed over time and across the care continuum, new types of provider partnerships are emerging in response. Physician practices need to consider options that include independence with risk-sharing arrangements, partnerships with other practices, acquisition by integrated systems/ ACOs— the choices will be numerous but the imperative will be effective positioning in order to be part of the clinical continuum that will attract patients and receive payments for care that are based on the new definitions of value. Systems will want to be affiliated with practices that can evidence excellence in quality, safety, patient experience and cost containment. Practices will want to make their partnering decisions on the same basis.

With regard to the financial goal of minimizing malpractice exposure and expense, effective patient engagement can play a significant role in improving a practice's risk profile. It is well known that ineffective physician communication, factors significantly into the decision to sue, as evidenced in study after study of malpractice claims. In one such study, for example, the top two reasons physicians were sued for malpractice were communication problems and inattention to the importance of a sound doctor-patient relationship. (Karp; Alaska Med Journal:2000; 42(2):48-9). Perhaps even more importantly, by engaging the patient, we will be helping the patient become as involved and as responsible as he or she truly should be. It will help with informed consent, patient compliance, and document that the patient is in control of many of the decisions and actions that sometimes lead to unfortunate adverse outcomes.

Q3: Do you see a role for technology in enhancing patient engagement, and if so, how?

Technology will play an important enabling role for patient engagement. In order for patients to engage, they need information. Today's consumers have become used to accessing all kinds of information electronically and have become quite adept at it. Patients are more informed than they have ever been, but still do not have access to all of the information they need to make good healthcare choices and participate in the management of their health. This information includes not only that related to provider selection and general information about health issues, but also the patient's own clinical information, to which they rightfully feel entitled.

The healthcare system is lagging in its responsiveness to these demands, but provider requirements at the federal level are giving new weight to this focus and the industry is moving more rapidly to deploy technology that will assist. EHRs are being adopted and patient portals that allow access to medical record information are becoming more commonplace. This not only provides patients access to information needed to better engage and participate in the care process, but also positions them to help the care team in their vigilance to ensure that things do not go wrong. As an example, patients can help monitor the follow-up on test results to mitigate against diagnostic error or ensure that information is transferred correctly to help in transitions across providers or settings.

One of the greatest opportunities may reside in the use of mobile technology to facilitate patient engagement. Over 80% of the population uses a mobile device and penetration is expected to continue to climb. There are tremendous opportunities associated with apps that patients can use before, during, and after healthcare encounters to assist them in their efforts to participate and at the same time provide efficiencies for the visit process that will accrue to the physician. As an example, patients can use apps to organize critical information in advance of an office visit, summarize questions they want to ask, and be prompted to ensure that they have current list of their medications. As these apps are developed, it will be important that they serve both the patient and the provider in order for them to become an inextricable part of the process.

Q4: How can a physician's practice move from patient engagement as a buzz word to actual enhanced patient engagement?

There are many things that a practice can do right now, beginning with an honest assessment of its practice culture to ensure that it is positioned for this important focus. Engagement often starts with the office staff, who must make the patient feel both welcomed and respected every time there is an encounter, either in person or over the phone. They should encourage the patient to ask questions and set the tone for clinical interactions that will occur with the physician. The physician must establish a culture in the practice that not only permits this, but encourages it. Staff must be treated with the same respect and care they are expected to show the patients and the culture must be one of transparency and learning for this to be the case.

There are many new methods emerging to move practices in this direction. They include ensuring that patient preference and values are solicited as part of the history and reflected in the design of the care plan; approaches to incorporating patients onto the care team; improved processes for appointment scheduling and follow-up between visits; using informed medical decision-making tools designed to include the patient in the care plan design; improved consenting processes and procedures that are more interactive and better at ensuring patient understanding of risk as well as benefit; and communication techniques to ensure patient comprehension of information. These are but of few of the strategies for moving practices in this direction. Importantly, early anecdotes indicate that paying more attention to patient engagement does not take more time in the long run, as it mitigates against time spent on avoidable and unnecessary follow-up of various kind.

Physician practices should also use existing survey tools to measure patient experience, which reflects effective patient engagement, and design improvement initiatives in response to the results.

Q5: Is patient engagement measurable, and if so, what is the best method?
We are at the early stages of both understanding the best approaches to activating and engaging patients as well as measuring the effectiveness of those approaches. There are methodologies for measuring patient activation (see Hibbard, et. al.) and for measuring patient experience of care, but not yet for measuring the level of engagement of individual patients or patient cohorts across practices. This is manifested in patient experience, however, which is beginning to be measured in a variety of ways, as previously mentioned, as it is incorporated into value-based payment schema. Scores and measure sets associated with CAHPS, VBMs, PQRS, MU— all are designed to both incent and measure better patient experience of care, which requires effective patient engagement. As with other measurement matters in healthcare during this time of change, proxy measures are being used to assess progress in patient engagement as well. Does a practice routinely ensure that patient preference is solicited and incorporated into care plans; does the practice survey its patients to ensure that the staff are responsive

and respectful and that the physician is welcoming of questions and provides adequate information to the patient; does the practice respect the role of the patient's family or advocate and ensure that they are included as desired by the patient; is there evidence of consenting practices that are interactive; does the practice use teach-back or other communication techniques—all of these are indicative of efforts to better engage patients and improve the relationships that are at the heart of the practice. More research and better measurement sets are indicated, but actually engaging one's patients is far more important than are the tools to measure it.

Ms. Pinakiewicz provides an excellent analysis and viewpoint of patient experience and engagement from the perspective of a national leader in patient safety. Next is a perspective from a national health policy expert.

Health Policy Expert: L. Gregory Pawlson, MD

Dr. Pawlson is the immediate past executive director for quality innovation for Blue Cross Blue Shield Association, Washington, DC. Prior to BCBSA, Dr. Pawlson was executive vice president of the National Committee for Quality Assurance (NCQA), where for over a decade he led the development of its research, measurement, and contracting activities, overseeing the ongoing development of the widely used HEDIS clinical performance measures. He also worked on the development of assessment programs for the Patient Centered Medical Homes and ACOs, and as liaison for NCQA to physician groups, including the AMA-led Physician Consortium for Practice Improvement, the American College of Physicians, the American Academy of Family Physicians and the American Academy of Pediatrics. He has held various directorship positions on health policy, including at the George Washington University Medical Center as director of the Institute for Health Policy, Outcomes and Human Values; as well as served as a Robert Wood Johnson Health Policy Fellow.

Q1: Patient satisfaction has recently transformed into the concept of "patient experience." How do you see that those two concepts differ?
Patient experience is a much broader, much more actionable concept than patient satisfaction. Satisfaction is a rather broad, highly subjective concept, and is greatly affected by how questions are framed, patient mood, and characteristics. Moreover, most clinicians see satisfaction ratings as a popularity contest unrelated to patient care. Finally, satisfaction is not directly actionable

(what change should a practice do to improve satisfaction) although it is often an important indicator of programs in the practice. Patient experience, on the other hand, can be very specific (did the doctor give you instructions you could understand?) and directly actionable (the practice or physician can make sure it provides every patient information that has been tested and shown to be understandable and useful). Everything that happens to patients when they are in a practice, from how they are greeted to how well the clinician listens to them, provides support and empathy, as well as makes a correct diagnosis and treatment, should be thought of as part of the patient experience of care.

> **Patient experience, on the other hand, can be very specific (did the doctor give you instructions you could understand?) and directly actionable (the practice or physician can make sure it provides every patient information that has been tested and shown to be understandable and useful).**

Q2: In your opinion, why should physician practices care about their patients' experiences with their practices?

For many reasons, but two particularly stand out with the premise that patients who have good experiences with the practice build up a layer of trust:

1. These patients are likely to stay with the practice even when insurers change as they frequently do, and will tell their friends and others about the practice; and

2. When something goes wrong, like a medical error, these patients are much less likely to sue.

If the practice not only builds trust with the patient by providing positive experiences over a long period of time, but then reinforces that by open and empathetic dialogue with the patient about a negative outcome and, if it was due to a medical error, by acknowledging the error, filing a malpractice claim is less likely, or if one is filed, it can be less likely to be successful. Of course, as the lawyers always tell me, acknowledgment of an error should be done by clinicians only after a thorough investigation of the matter and with the aid and support of hospital risk management and/or a lawyer experienced in these matters.

Q3: What's different today about the patient experience than perhaps 5 or 10 years ago?

Consumers, including those who participate in healthcare as patients, are demanding more information and better overall service from nearly every kind of service provider, including healthcare. Moreover, those who pay for healthcare, whether patients themselves, the government, or private employers, are demanding more accountability for quality and safety from providers. This is combined with a reimbursement environment that is continuing to move towards payment based on performance and quality rather than just on the volume of services.

Q4: Do you find that physician practices across the country are truly embracing the concept of patient experience? And if so, what are the characteristics of a practice that has been able to successfully do so?

Many practices are taking a very proactive and constructive approach to improving the patient experience of care. These practices are characterized by thoughtful, progressive leadership; engaged staff; and the identification and implementation of "best in class" processes and practices not only from medicine, but from other service providers as well, similar to the five-star service program described in this book.

Q5: How do you see the patient engagement concept impacting physicians and their practices in the future?

Patient engagement is a set of principles and processes that in most cases directly and positively impact not only the patient experience of care, but also influence the outcomes of care, especially in persons who have serious chronic illnesses. There is a substantial and growing literature that shows that patient behaviors, including things like adherence to treatments including medication, are strongly influenced by how engaged and involved they feel they are in decision making and the intervention itself. Greater patient engagement in both their own treatment, as well as in how the practice functions overall, appear to have a positive impact on patient retention by the practice, and in some pay-for-performance or global payment programs, my also lead to positive financial impact. Finally, and perhaps more importantly, physician enjoyment of their practices is usually bolstered by having most patients engaged in an active way with the practice.

The commentary from Diane Pinakiewicz and Dr. Pawlson make clear that there is a need for a culture change in healthcare delivery that embraces the physician-patient engagement concept. It can be of greater value today and into the future for patients, clinicians, health payors, and medical professional liability insurers. All the stakeholder interests are aligned.

For the healthcare providers, patient engagement can:

- Enhance practice morale;
- Decrease time spent on patient complaints; and
- Reduce professional liability risk.

For patients, the obvious impact can be improvement in health outcomes and overall patient health. Health payors benefit in enhanced visit efficiency and of course patient health, reducing the costs of healthcare. The medical professional liability insurers can benefit from reduced number of adverse events that otherwise are the basis for costly lawsuits.

Patient engagement is really going beyond "patient satisfaction" and the "patient experience of care." Patient satisfaction is a result of how a patient *feels*. It is a difficult measure to meet, as what satisfies one patient is different than what might satisfy another; worse yet, being a satisfied patient does not necessarily correlate with reasonableness. For example, a patient may be dis-satisfied with how long he had to wait in the waiting room for his appointment; yet, if he arrived early and expected to be seen early, the practice is not going to be able to satisfy him. Patient experience of care goes a step further to evaluating how a patient *perceives* his interactions with the providers and practice. Patient engagement really goes beyond requiring *interaction* of patients with their providers and becoming part of the care team. Doing so will often affect patient satisfaction and patient experience of care scores, but truly is an entirely more robust concept— one that is part of a true five-star service culture.

Engaging with patients means clinicians need to be able to communicate with their patients, understand their values and desires, and their ethnicity. In the next chapter, we explore these potential challenges, and suggest that clinicians will need to focus more in these areas in order to truly accomplish patient engagement.

CHAPTER 8

A Highlight on Cultural Competency

(with contribution from Lisa Eng, DO[1])

The clinicians' role in patient care post-ACA, has transformed; no longer will physicians be able to treat the disease without knowing or understanding their patient and be successful with their practice at the same time. The post-ACA reimbursement strategies and care collaboration strategies will make it more difficult for physicians to "operate" in a silo. The oft-cited example of tunnel-vision care is the surgeon who says, "I'm a surgeon. I do surgery. That's it. That's what I do— surgery. I do not interact with the patient." That approach will not work for the long-term. Interaction is needed in order to enhance patient outcomes through patient engagement, and that interaction must be *meaningful*.

To be meaningful, the providers and the patients need to not only communicate, but also be on the same page about care plans. This is best accomplished by developing care plans in concert with the patient, incorporating the patient's values and culture. Progressively this will become more important as cultural diversity continues to expand in the United States.

A term you have probably heard, but may not have paid much attention to, is "cultural competence." The U.S. Department of Health & Human Services defines "cultural competence" as:

> Cultural and linguistic competence is a set of congruent behaviors, attitudes, and policies that come together in a system, agency, or among professionals that enables effective work in cross-cultural situations. 'Culture' refers to integrated patterns of human behavior

that include the language, thoughts, communications, actions, customs, beliefs, values, and institutions of racial, ethnic, religious, or social groups. 'Competence' implies having the capacity to function effectively as an individual and an organization within the context of the cultural beliefs, behaviors, and needs presented by consumers and their communities.[2]

It seems like common sense: To be effective requires working within the realm of patient values and cultures and unique health and behavior characteristics of a cultural group. Yet, it is not the norm.

According to the most recent study published by the Agency for Healthcare Research and Quality (AHRQ),[3]

- Healthcare quality and access to care is suboptimal, particularly for minority and low-income groups; and
- Disparities in care are not changing.

The study addresses disparities in care, access, and treatment, and sets forth examples of worsening disparities. Disparities are worsening in the African American population compared to the White population in number of maternal deaths per 100,000 live births.[4] Data show that infants born to African American women are 1.5 to 3 times more likely to die than those born to women of other races/ethnicities.[5] Disparities are worsening in the Asian population compared to the White population in adjusted incidence of end-stage renal disease due to diabetes per million population.[6] These are just a few examples.

Additional data reports disparities that include:

- American Indian and Alaska Native infants die from SIDS at nearly 2.5 times the rate of White infants.[7]
- African Americans, American Indians, and Alaska Natives are 2 times more likely to have diabetes in comparison to Whites.[8]
- Hispanic women are more than 1.5 times as likely to be diagnosed with cervical cancer. The Vietnamese experience the highest invasive cervical cancer incidence.[9]
- African Americans, American Indians, and Alaska Natives are twice as likely to have diabetes as Whites.[10]
- Hispanics are 1.5 times more likely than non-Hispanic Whites to die from diabetes.[11]

- African Americans have a 5-year survival rate for all cancers of 53% compared to 64% for Whites.[12]

With increasing racial and ethnic communities and linguistic groups, predictions include that by 2050, half of the U.S. population will be comprised of racial and ethnic minorities. That prediction, combined with the new healthcare environment focus on quality, safety, increased access of care, and reduced costs (national health care reform), makes a focus on cultural competency more important than ever.

With increasing racial and ethnic communities and linguistic groups, predictions include that by 2050, half of the U.S. population will be comprised of racial and ethnic minorities. That prediction, combined with the new healthcare environment focus on quality, safety, increased access of care, and reduced costs (national health care reform), makes a focus on cultural competency more important than ever. Its benefits can include:[13]

- Better adherence to medical treatment plans;
- Better outcomes;
- Increased respect and mutual understanding;
- Increased participation by patients in their own healthcare;
- Decreased costs; and
- Enhanced patient satisfaction.[14]

Studies have shown a relationship between limited-English-proficiency (LEP)[15] patients and adverse events. For example, The Joint Commission published results indicating[16]:

- LEP patients are much more likely than English-proficient patients to suffer an adverse event where the provider's action or lack of it causes unintentional harm to the patient (49.1% v. 29.5%);

- LEP patients are more likely (52.4%) than English-proficient patients (35.9%) to suffer adverse events related to communication errors (52.4% v. 35.9%); and
- LEP patient events involving harm tend to also be more injurious or harmful than those involving non-LEP patients (46.8% v. 24.4%).

Adverse events involving an injury are 100% of medical malpractice claims, as every medical malpractice lawsuit necessarily involves an adverse event with injury. Therefore, by enhancing cultural competency, you can favorably impact liability risk. Note that issues involving cultural competency and LEP are also the types of factors that can affect whether a lawsuit is filed or the value of a lawsuit. It is often more difficult to defend a case involving poor or ineffective communication, or a failure to obtain assistance services for an LEP patient. Most juries simply are not forgiving when it comes to these types of issues.

Further, one study found that 27% of LEP patients who need but do not receive a professional interpreter in a medical setting report not understanding their medication instructions, compared with only 2% of patients who either do not need an interpreter or who need and receive one.

Accordingly, addressing LEP barriers can decrease liability risk and enhance patient outcomes.

Consider another economic benefit that can be derived from enhanced cultural competency: an opportunity to enhance market share and retain patients. The reality is that many culturally distinct populations are underserved, which provides an opportunity for physicians who want to engage with these populations, and do so effectively. For example, the Asian population in Brooklyn and New York City have benefitted from focused resources where doctors speak the patients' language and are actually part of the culture. Doctors wishing to tap into this market will not only attempt to speak Chinese or Korean, but will hire people who speak the language and modify their business to accommodate this profitable and captive market. Such opportunities exist not only in the large cities, but smaller ones as well. Perhaps the most important point here is the value such arrangements provide to quality patient care and outcomes.

The need to understand the "language" or idioms of the patient, knowing whom your patient considers an authority, being aware of all barriers and beliefs that will promote or impede a patient's compliance with recommended testing and treatment, will ultimately give your patient the best chance at good outcomes, including participation in their own healthcare, and consequently their exposure. These concepts are going to become more important through time.

In healthcare, there are more opportunities than you might realize to enhance cultural competency. It should be considered in your brochures, materials, and other resources; your communications; and in certain important documents, such as patient discharge instructions, intake forms related to important health concerns, and consent forms. In fact, HHS guidance indicates that meaningful access for LEP patients to "vital" documents is necessary. Know your patient population and have certain key documents translated into the languages of relevance to your patient population.

Here are some tips to enhance cultural competency in your practice:

- Understand that culturally, people may have other treatment regiments, and these may interact with more traditional remedies; inquire about these regiments. Ask your patients to bring in a list of their remedies.
- Understand your specific patient population demographics and focus your cultural competency efforts accordingly.
- Focus on key "vital" documents and have prepared templates of these documents in non-English languages you most often encounter at your practice.
- Have a cultural competency policy in place for your practice, setting the expectations among your staff.
- Provide education for your specific patient population; perhaps coordinate with your local hospital.
- Conduct a "cultural competence" survey of your practice (see example).

We are not suggesting an overhaul of your practice, but rather enhancements to your current five-star culture by assuring cultural competence within your practice, not only for the benefit of your patients, but also your. Again, with the focus post-ACA on patient quality of care and outcomes and a move away from fee-for-service to linking quality to reimbursement, and the link of patient satisfaction/experience of care to reimbursement, cultural competency is another tool that can affect outcomes and patient satisfaction/experience of care.

Evaluate Your Cultural Competency[17]

Check the box if the answer to the statement is True.

Physical Environment, Materials, and Other Resources

☐ My office displays posters, pictures, and other materials that reflect the cultures and ethnic backgrounds of the patients served by my practice.

☐ We provide magazines, brochures, and other printed materials in the reception areas that reflect the different cultures served by our practice.

☐ When using videos, films, DVDs, or other media resources, I assure that they reflect the cultures of the patients served by our practice.

Communication Style

☐ I attempt to learn and use key words of the language of patients if other than English, so that I may better communicate with them and engage with them.

☐ When appropriate, I use visual aids and/or drawings to enhance communication with patients who are of limited English proficiency.

☐ Our practice has a written policy and procedure regarding use of interpreters with limited English proficiency.

☐ My staff includes bilingual or multi-lingual individuals.

☐ When possible, I provide written care instructions to patients of limited English proficiency in their dominant language.

Values and Attitude

☐ I avoid imposing values that may conflict with or be inconsistent with those of cultures or ethnic groups other than my own.

☐ Our practice has a strict policy forbidding use of racial and ethnic slurs.

☐ I accept and respect that male-female roles in families may vary significantly among different cultures (who makes the major decisions for the family, for example).

☐ I understand that religion, spirituality, and other beliefs may influence how patients and their families respond to illness, death, disability, and disease.

☐ I keep abreast of new developments in care and treatment as they relate to racial and ethnic groups.

References

1. Brief biographical sketch: Lisa Eng, D.O. is a board-certified, practicing ob-gyn in Brooklyn, NY. She has a strong interest in enhancing cultural competency in health care. She has chaired the task force for cultural competency for ACOG/District II and is a member of the Medical Society of the State of New York's Committee to Eliminate Healthcare Disparities. She is the past president of the Association of Chinese American Physicians and Chinese Community Accountable Care Organization. She is a board member of the New York State Osteopathic Medical Society, immediate past president of the Medical Society of the County of Kings and Bay Ridge Medical Society. She is also president of Patients First Co-op.

2. See http://minorityhealth.hhs.gov (citing Cross, 1989).

3. 2012 National Healthcare Quality Report. U.S. Department of Health and Human Services. Agency for Healthcare Research and Quality. Publication No. 13-0002, May 2013 (accessible at www.ahrq.gov/rsearch/findings/nhqrdr/index.html).

4. 2012 National Healthcare Quality Report. U.S. Department of Health and Human Services. Agency for Healthcare Research and Quality. Publication No. 13-0002, May 2013 (accessible at www.ahrq.gov/rsearch/findings/nhqrdr/index.html).

5. See: http://www.cdc.gov/mmwr/preview/mmwrhtml/su6001a1.htm and http://www.who.int/sdhconference/background/news/facts/en/

6. 2012 National Healthcare Quality Report. U.S. Department of Health and Human Services. Agency for Healthcare Research and Quality. Publication No. 13-0002, May 2013 (accessible at www.ahrq.gov/rsearch/findings/nhqrdr/index.html).

7. See http://minorityhealth.hhs.gov/templates/content.aspx?ID=3038

8. See http://www.sophe.org/sophe/PDF/2000_Resolution%20for%20Eliminating%20Racial%20and%20Ethnic%20Health%20Disparities.pdf

9. See http://crchd.cancer.gov/about/examples.html and http://www.cancer.org/acs/groups/content/@nho/documents/document/ffhispanicslatinos20092011.pdf

10. See http://minorityhealth.hhs.gov/templates/browse.aspx?lvl=3&lvlid=62

11. See http://clinical.diabetesjournals.org/content/30/3/130.full and http://minorityhealth.hhs.gov/templates/browse.aspx?lvl=3&lvlid=62

12. See http://www.cancer.org/acs/groups/content/@nho/documents/document/cffaa20092010pdf.pdf

13. Wilson-Stronks A., Mutha S. From the perspective of CEOs: What motivates hospitals to embrace cultural competence. *J. of Healthcare Management.* 55 (2010) 339-352.

14. See Cultural Competence in Health Care: Is It Important for People with Chronic Conditions? Center on an Aging Society. Georgetown Univ. 2004 *citing* Cooper LA, Roter DL. Patient-provider communication: The effect of race and ethnicity on process and outcomes of healthcare. In *Unequal treatment: confronting racial and ethnic disparities in health care* (pp. 552-593) Washington, DC: The National Academies Press.

15. According to the 2012 U.S. Census Bureau, over 60 million individuals speak a language other than English (21% of the population), and 25 million of those speak English less than "very well U.S. Census

Bureau 2012 . Profile of selected social characteristics (Table DP02 and Table CP02) (accessible at http://factfinder2.census.gov) (last accessed 9/27/13).

16. Chandrika Divi et al., "Language proficiency and adverse Events in U.S. hospitals: A pilot study," International Journal for Quality in Health Care. 2007. 19(2): 60–67.

17. Adapted from the National Center for Cultural Competence Self –Assessment Checklist for Personnel Providing Behavioral Health and Supports to Children, Youth and their Families (accessible at http://www.georgetown.edu/research/gucchd/nccc/documents/checklistbehavioralhealth.pdf).

CHAPTER 9

Perspectives: Real-Life Commentary on Successes and Barriers

One of our goals in writing this book is to provide healthcare professionals with practical information on five-star service. In this chapter, we provide you with real-life, current commentary on successes and barriers to a five-star culture— from various perspectives: an academic-affiliated surgical practice; an Ob/Gyn practice of 11 healthcare professionals; a community-based hospital; and a primary care practice.

Perspective of a University-Affiliated, Hospital-Based Surgeon

Steven Schwaitzberg, MD, is a board-certified surgeon working at Cambridge Health Alliance. Cambridge, MA, where his general surgery department took the initiative to impact its patient experience of care by thinking outside the box, with an understanding of its patients and other factors affecting survey response rates. He writes:

Every practice has unique features that describe the challenges and opportunities in providing and improving care. For our multi-specialty surgery clinics charged with the responsibility of improving the patient experience of care (PEOC), as measured by one of the well-known survey instruments, we felt stymied. Our university-affiliated, community-based hospital also serves as a safety net institution for the region. This dramatically drives up the number of non-English-speaking patients whom we care for. Commercial ambulatory surveys are printed in English and do not capture patients from our top six other languages (Spanish, Portuguese, Haitian-Creole, Mandarin, Bengali, or Hindi).

In addition, these commercial surveys are often quite long and detailed. It should be no surprise that our return rate on the surveys mailed to the patients' homes was a dismal 4%. There is really not much you can do to impact PEOC with a return rate so poor. The numbers fluctuated dramatically since a few responses in either direction could produce wide variations in the "results."

Our general surgery division chief, Ketan Sheth, devised a simple and ingenious plan. He felt we were asking too many questions, not to mention often in the wrong languages. Internally we devised a one-question survey. It was not difficult to have our interpreter service translate this into many languages: The question was:

"Please tell us ONE thing that would have made your appointment better today."

We provided space for the anonymous response on the same sheet. Unlike the commercial surveys that were mailed to the peoples' homes, this survey question was given in the clinic in the appropriate language, and with the interpreters available to help the patients formulate their responses. As they left the office, the patients placed the completed surveys in a box.

The survey is now sent out each season for a two-week period to hundreds of general surgery patients. To our amazement, return rates range from 41% to 67%. The most pleasant surprise was that the vast majority (~75%) thought their visits were excellent. However, those numbers do not form an impetus for improvement. So we reviewed the negative responses and identified a few major themes.

Our negative response rate went down from 23% to 8% in three survey periods.

First and foremost is the issue of timeliness on the part of the doctor. Second was the issue of parking (which in our population is a concern about spending available cash despite the fact that parking fees in the downtown tertiary centers is far more expense). The two are somewhat interconnected, as a long delay in being seen by the doctor adds to the parking fees.

Armed with this insight, we targeted our efforts at template accuracy and keeping patients informed about the wait if the surgeon was behind schedule and asking if there was anything (like a glass of water or a cup of coffee) we could do in extreme cases. We also posted a sign in our waiting room that stated: "If you have been waiting more than 15 minutes for your appointment, please notify our receptionist. Thank you."

Our negative response rate went down from 23% to 8% in three survey periods.

Clearly, large survey instruments are here to stay and will likely be tied to reimbursement. The lesson here, for us, was that we saw we needed to do something outside of the CMS survey in order to obtain truly useful information to impact our PEOC the way we desired—with an inexpensive, statistically unproven homemade survey in multiple languages.

Steven D. Schwaitzberg, MD
Chief of Surgery
Cambridge Health Alliance
Cambridge, MA

Perspective of a Physician-Office Based OB-Gyn

Richard Waldman, MD, is a practicing Ob-Gyn at the Associates for Women's Medicine in Syracuse, NY. He is past president of the American College of Obstetricians & Gynecologists (2010-2011) and has been involved in many leadership positions at the regional and the national levels. Dr. Waldman began his own practice as a single Ob/Gyn and a midwife. Today, his practice is comprised of 10 physicians, 6 non-physician professionals, and over 100 employees. He serves as president of that group, Associates for Women's Medicine. He is also president of the medical staff at St. Joseph's Hospital Health Center and a member of the Board of Trustees. He previously served as the hospital's chairman for the department of Ob/Gyn and medical director of performance improvement. He shares:

Our practice has always viewed patient satisfaction as a critical success factor. We had done crude patient satisfaction surveys for many years. At a monthly quality meeting, we review every complaint, problem, or near-miss that occurs.

We are now of the thinking that we must move beyond patient satisfaction to respect and patient engagement. Our goal is 100% patient satisfaction with their experience of care with us. Our motivation is enhancing clinical results, with the belief that patient-centered care leads to better-engaged patients and better outcomes. Of course today there is also a financial incentive that is gaining ground, related to this metric.

We believe we can meet our goal with the help of a new patient experience survey platform. I was recently involved in evaluating an obstetric-specific physician practice specific patient experience survey, which I know is mentioned earlier in this book. I found the survey to be uniquely focused on obstetrical patient experiences, which will provide our group with truly actionable metrics to reach our goal.

RICHARD WALDMAN, MD
Associates for Women's Medicine
Syracuse, NY

Camden Clark Medical Center is a 248-bed, not-for-profit, acute care facility in Parkersburg, WV. The Center is committed to the patient experience of care, with support coming from the top of the organization. For several years it has had a patient experience leader, Mandy Foley, RN, whose job it is to evaluate and impact the patient experience of care in collaboration with the leadership and staff. The team took a deep dive into their HCAHPS scores, with a desire to impact their OB department scores. Here is their story.

One of the first things our team did in our quest to improve the patient experience was to look at our Press Ganey scores, specifically the questions that seemed to have the highest correlation with "overall rating" and "would you recommend." Unlike other units in the hospital, room appearance, cleanliness, and pleasantness of room decor consistently proved to be a high priority for our Ob/Gyn population. We also recognized that the Ob/Gyn population had a higher dissatisfaction rate when it came to discharge education.

When looking at the room appearance, we reviewed patient comments from our patient satisfaction surveys and also spoke with our patients in order to gain more feedback. We found that patients were generally very pleased with our delivery rooms, which had recently been renovated and are very spacious with hardwood floors and newer amenities. However, once our mothers delivered and were moved to the post-partum unit, they became dissatisfied. While all private rooms, the post-partum rooms are much smaller, with outdated décor that is hospital-like in appearance.

The rooms were stark white, the portraits were all very outdated, and the only lighting consisted of overhead bright florescent lights. After much literature review, the team found information on evidence-based practices regarding the best environment for newborns and their mothers. After birth, it is best to have a calming environment that induces relaxation and bonding for a newborn and his or her mother. This environment includes warm colors, low-level lighting to encourage babies to open their eyes and see their mother, as well as an inviting and comforting environment that makes a mother feel more like she is in her nursery at home. All of these strategies help put a mother and baby at ease and can have many benefits such as better milk let down and enhanced bonding.

To help promote employee engagement, we let our professional practice council help with the selection process in choosing the changes for our post-partum rooms. We decided to paint the rooms in a soft taupe color to help provide the warm, calm, and relaxing environment we were seeking. With the help of a local modern photographer, we opted to replace the outdated portraits in the rooms with modern-style photos of local newborns on large canvases. We have these canvas prints in all the post-partum rooms and throughout the entire OB department. We replaced the privacy curtains in the room with a much more modern home-like material that is a warm sage color. Two wall sconces were placed at the head of the patient's bed to allow for the low-level lighting and to also add to the modern home-like feel that we were aiming for.

Last but not least, in regards to the atmosphere of the room, we had all of our rooms deep cleaned, the floors waxed, wall boards placed to prevent future damage from moving carts/beds, and adjustments to our heating and cooling units to provide a more comfortable and clean environment. With all of these cosmetic changes to our post-partum rooms, we immediately began to see a rise in some of our patient satisfaction scores.

Of course, these changes did not come about without challenges. First, we had to develop a case for our department's wants/needs to sell to our leadership team because all of these changes, obviously, had a cost associated with them. After much consideration, our project funding was approved and we were on to the exciting part of designing our rooms. We worked with our engineering depart-ment to develop a plan of how and when each of the rooms would be completed. The most challenging part of the whole renovation was figuring out how to take a room out of use in order to complete its renovations. We have an extremely busy OB department and deliver an average of 130 babies per month. Having only 13 beds in our post-partum department often times created a bed crunch for us and we would have to postpone renovations until our census dropped a bit. The entire renovation project took eight months to complete. This has been somewhat frustrating for us because we have not yet been able to see the full impact on our patient satisfaction scores. While there has been an increase in our measures, we are eagerly awaiting our patient satisfactions scores to come in since the project's completion (which just finished up in the first week of April 2014). So far, our HCAHPS cleanliness score has jumped 6%.

Looking at our discharge education, we realized that our current method of education is outdated. We also did a lot of literature review and research on educational materials specific for obstetric patients. Given that our average OB patient is typically 16–35 years old, we understood that our method of education needed to be geared towards that age group. Previously, we used handouts, booklets, and VHS videos to help us deliver education to our new moms and their families. However, this particular generation is technologically savvy and thrives on receiving information immediately via Internet resources.

We looked into several different commonly advertised television/Internet education systems for patients that were amazing; however, we just did not have a budget to incorporate any of those systems at the time. We worked closely with our IT team to create our own education system with the use of Smart TVs. As a unit, we determined what modern videos would meet the needs of our patients best and got the copyrights for those videos and had them uploaded to our televisions. Patients can watch the education on demand at their convenience. The videos will also be posted on the hospital website so parents can access the information from home. Also, having Internet available on the Smart TVs allows patients to browse the Internet for other resources and also gives our patients another method to stay connected with their friends and family while in the hospital. Another benefit of the Smart TVs is that we can upload new videos very easily.

As for barriers, it was expected to take six weeks to have our Smart TVs up and running . . . however, the televisions were on back order for six months. In the last few weeks of spring 2014, all of our flat screen TVs have been installed and the Smart TV function should be up and operating in a few weeks. We are hopeful that replacing our old 19" box televisions with 37" flat screens Smart

TVs will help to improve some of our patient satisfaction scores as well as patient engagement. We are excited to see the impact that our fully completed renovations will have on our patients!

Of course, patient satisfaction involves much more than just the look and feel of a room. As we do more and more literature review to find best practices, we recognize that there are always opportunities to create better quality care and experiences for our patients. Some of our next steps will be challenging as we are working to change our model of nursing care. This will prove to be a challenging yet exciting experience!

MARTHA DAWSON, RN, BSN
Director of Women's and Children's Services
Camden Clark Medical Center
Parkersburg, WV

So many of the cultures we encouraged and practiced in five-star service are also key to the success of a patient centered medical home office.

Perspective of a Physician Office Practice Manager

A primary care practice of 16 physicians began a journey up the five-star service curve eight years ago, before the post-ACA concepts of patient experience of care, tied to reimbursement, and the patient centered medical home. At the time, the impetus was really about enhancing the physician-patient relationship to achieve benefits of better patient outcomes and reduced liability risk. As it turns out, the practice's five-star journey is paving the way to the patient centered medical home. Lois Summers, practice manager for the group, explains:

Creating a five-star service culture began at General Internal Medicine of Lancaster in 2005. Now it seems long ago, but in some ways like only yesterday. So many of the cultures we encouraged and practiced in five-star service are also key to the success of a patient centered medical home office. Five-star is service excellence every day with each and every contact. True service excellence leaves a positive fingerprint on all we do, not just for the patient but as a team working together. By practicing five-star service, we developed many helpful behaviors and attitudes that become contagious and served to help us as we now work toward treating the whole patient and addressing all needs at each visit. Providers, staff, and patients, participate in the care of the whole patient. Five-star was the stepping stone to the patient centered care we provide our patients today. Like 5 Star, Patient Centered Care puts the patient at the center of the care.

LOIS SUMMERS, MANAGER

General Internal Medicine of Lancaster

Division of Physician's Alliance Limited

Lancaster, PA

Fifty-Eight Five-Star Hints

1. Be an example for your colleagues.
2. Use a five-star attestation form (Figure 3-2) with all new hires.
3. Provide all personnel who communicate on the phone with telephone etiquette training.
4. Keep automated voice systems to fewer than six prompts.
5. Answer all calls within three rings.
6. Ask for permission of callers before putting a caller on hold.
7. Return calls and messages within one business day.
8. Keep patients informed of any delays in the waiting room, on the phone, in the exam room.
9. Smile! (Even when it hurts.)
10. Post a sign inviting patients to inform the check-in desk if they are waiting more than 15 minutes past their appointment time.
11. When dealing with difficult patients, take 10 seconds before responding.
12. Empathize with patients *and their families*.
13. Treat your co-workers with respect.
14. Survey your employees on an annual basis to learn their thoughts about the practice environment.
15. Be your brother's keeper . . . constructive criticism is good.
16. Have a written patient complaint policy that includes the roles and responsibilities of staff.
17. Create a mission statement, value statement, and employee promise, and post them visibly at the practice, on marketing materials, and on your website.
18. Create a patient portal that allows patients confidential access to their medical records.
19. Slow down . . . do not *appear* rushed to patients and staff.
20. Always introduce yourself to the patient.
21. Actively listen!
22. Avoid negative body language, including:

- Crossing arms
- Hands on hips
- Rolling eyes

23. Tell a co-worker about any poor five-star habits.
24. Sit down or stand up to be at eye level with your patient when holding a conversation.
25. Remember patient privacy; hold conversations about patient health information behind closed doors.
26. View your patient as a person, not solely as a disease or medical condition.
27. Be punctual—for the start of the work day, every day.
28. Get some one-on-one coaching from a professional five-star trainer (if needed).
29. Think incrementally; focus on one five-star change at a time.
30. Never use profane language at the office.
31. Don't let technology issues get to you. Call on someone for assistance.
32. Gather, evaluate, and benchmark your practice's patient experience data.
33. Publish five-star fixes to your staff.
34. Make eye contact with your patients.
35. Assure your exam rooms, waiting room, file room, bathroom, and the like are clean and organized.
36. Hold a monthly drawing for patients; invite them to enter at the time of check out from the office.
37. Escort patients from the exam room to the check out.
38. Provide patients with a $5 gift card to a local food establishment, for referrals, with a hand-written note of thanks.
39. Have up-to-date magazines and newspapers available in the waiting room.
40. Put "five-star" on your board agenda— near the top!
41. Try to "rehab" the naysayers, but when it's clear it isn't going to work, don't keep them!
42. Assure the office is free of clutter in hallways.
43. Explain the exam process to patients as you are going through the exam.
44. Provide patients with written instructions on their care plan at the end of the appointment.
45. Provide annual education to staff on five-star service, incorporating tips and tools they can use.

46. Greet patients by their name.
47. Assure that all staff have clearly visible name tags with not only their name, but also their position.
48. Keep personal conversations to a minimum.
49. Incorporate systems that allow patients to speak with a physician after hours regarding emergency matters.
50. Recognize special patient populations that may require understandings that can affect your approach in patient relationship building, such as underweight/overweight patients; the elderly; those with varying religious beliefs or values; the hearing impaired; those with language differences. Avoid insensitivities and provide reasonable accommodations.
51. Identify barriers to five-star service and address them.
52. Hire a shadow patient to delve into the patient experience.
53. Use your patient complaints as a source of information to improve the patient experience.
54. Provide staff with scripts as a tool to support them in their contact with patients.
55. Recognize that *every* patient contact counts.
56. Have a policy on reporting normal *and* abnormal test results to patients.
57. When things go wrong, do not prejudge or make conclusions without all the facts.
58. Assess your own five-star skills and when you identify weaknesses, look for solutions.

CME/Quiz

1. All of the following are established benefits of five-star customer service, except:
   a. Reduced liability risk
   b. A better working environment
   c. Less interaction with patients
   d. Higher patient satisfaction
2. T/F Physicians do not need to worry about HCAHPS. It is something for the hospital to worry about.
   a. True
   b. False
3. The concept of five-star includes:
   a. A focus on quality care
   b. Patient interactions with your practice
   c. Internal five star
   d. All of the above.
4. T/F Examples of true five-star service are prevalent in physician medical practices.
   a. True
   b. False
5. Which of the following identifies the step-by-step plan for a five-star plan as discussed in this book?
   a. Create a five-star committee, get leadership buy-in, develop a 1- 3- 5-year plan, educate staff.
   b. Obtain leadership buy-in, create a 1- 3- 5-year plan, kick-off to staff, create a five-star committee.
   c. Create a five-star committee, prepare a 1- 3- 5-year plan, get leadership buy-in, educate staff.
   d. Obtain leadership buy-in, establish a five-star committee, kick-off your five-star culture program to staff, create a 1- 3- 5-year plan.

6. Internal five-star is best described by which statement below?
   a. Internal five-star is about how the practice treats patients.
   b. Internal five-star is about how everyone in the practice treats one another, even in times of stress.
   c. Internal five-star means evaluating your colleagues' behavior and telling them to change.
7. Which one of the following was included in this book as an example of a practice event that can detract from the patient relationship?
   a. Difficulty obtaining a refill
   b. Patients overhearing staff and physicians arguing
   c. The inability to reach a physician by phone "after hours"
   d. A messy waiting room.
8. All of the following are part of the post-adverse event continuity, except:
   a. Empathy
   b. Five-star
   c. Loyalty
   d. Confrontation
9. T/F When it comes to "disclosing an error," research suggests patients want to be told about the error, understand what happened and why, know any consequences will be mitigated, be assured future recurrences will be prevented, and have emotional support.
   a. True
   b. False
10. Cultural competency is important to the five-star concept because:
    a. Everyone should just be able to speak their patients' language.
    b. Cultural competency can enhance the patient experience.
    c. Cultural competency means your patients should conform to your cultural values in order to enhance their experience.
    d. Cultural competency is not important to the five-star concept.

Answer Key

1. C; 2. B; 3. D; 4. B; 5. D; 6. B; 7. B; 8. D; 9. B; 10. B

Tools and Forms

www.ingramcontent.com/pod-product-compliance
Lightning Source LLC
Chambersburg PA
CBHW061608220326
41598CB00024BC/3495